This book didn't start out to be this book. I'd originally sent my wonderful then-editor at Alyson, Scott Brassart, a proposal to edit an anthology of queer men's writings about their favorite kinks—essays somewhere between abstruse theoretical musings and self-indulgent confessional blat. When Scott suggested I write the whole damn thing myself, I was a bit taken aback.

"I'm not the kinkiest guy in town," I protested. "I'm not the sexiest guy in town. Hell, I'm not even the best-hung guy in town…not quite."

"That's OK," Scott said.

"Yeah, but who's going to want to read about the erotic exploits of someone they've never heard of?"

"Readers have heard of you," Scott said. "And the rest of what you said is why you'd be just the right person to do the book."

Listen, I don't know about the rest of you, but when someone says to me "Go write a book and we'll publish it," I tend to take notice. So I signed the contract.

As I went to work putting all this sleazy stuff on paper, I came to realize that what I was doing—fraught with the queasy joys of self-exposure—was a bit risky. You see, I have no idea, dear reader, who you are or what you'll think of all this.

I'm not much of a joiner or a true believer, so if you're a committed member of one scene or another you may find me slightly, oh, cheeky. But then nobody hired me to be a booster for perversion. So let me say this right out front: I don't claim to have the last word on anything. This book is not comprehensive, nor was it intended to be. I'm sure there'll be lots of men just aching to correct me on one point or another. That's fine, but don't assume that because we differ on nomenclature, philosophy, whatever, that I'm just a wanker. I'm not, OK?

If, on the other hand, you're curious but largely inexperienced, you may find this book scary or vaguely discouraging. Well, I can't pretend that slapping some guy around to get your sexual jollies is an unmixed bag, all sunshine and flowers. It shouldn't be, and it ain't.

And if you suspect you're one of the men in the book, rest assured that I've disguised your identity, changing enough details so only you and I will know for sure. (Unless you're one of the brave and exhibitionistic fellows who said "Use my real name. Please." Even then, I didn't name you—sorry—but I have kept you semi-identifiable. Lucky you.)

Whoever you are, I'm hoping you find my diaries of the journey worth the reading: that every once in a while you'll think *Wow! I've felt just like that!* Or *Hmm…I never thought about fist fucking quite that way before.* Or *Gee, that spanking stuff sounds like fun. Maybe I'll give it a try.* Maybe, even, my description of one scene or another might prompt you to jack off. That'd be nice. And if you someday meet up with me, please be gentle. Listen, I was thinking of subtitling this book *You'll Never Fuck Ass in This Town Again.* So be nice. Or nasty. As the case may be.

As *Kinkorama* took shape, I realized that, rather than writing a how-to or an I-know-it-all book, I was creating something of a travelogue: Here are the places I've been, here's how they felt, here's what I thought about them. It's just that the "places" were spots such as under the boot of a handsome, nasty German; in a tied-up guy's butt; or at a party devoted to tickle torture. *Lonely Planet* meets Krafft-Ebing.

Since I embarked on my writing career, I've had the fortune to meet a number of folks who are not just excellent authors, but also sex-radical activists who put themselves on the line for the cause of libidinal freedom. This book is dedicated to three of the best, who've taught me much about fearlessness: Patrick Califia, the late Scott O'Hara, and Dr. Carol Queen.

And to William.

CONTENTS

FOREWORD ♦ xi

INTRODUCTION: I Like to Do *That*? ♦ 1

1 Satori in the Men's Room:
Glory Holes and Bathroom Sex ♦ 7

2 Just Looking, Thanks:
Exhibitionism, Voyeurism, and Three-Ways ♦ 17

3 This Little Piggy: Foot Fetishism ♦ 31

4 Lending a Hand:
Fisting and Other Extreme Sex ♦ 43

5 Sticks and Stone: Verbal Abuse ♦ 55

6 Acting With Restraint: Bondage ♦ 67

7 Ouch! Pain Play ♦ 77

8 Welcome to the Woodshed:
Punishment Scenes ♦ 91

9 This Way to the Ninth Circle:
S/M Play Parties ♦ 105

10 Doing It in the Road:
Street Fairs and Shamelessness ♦ 121

11 Macho, Macho Man:
Leather Contests and Other Butch Pursuits ♦ 135

12 That's SIR to You: Masters and Slaves ♦ 145

13 Gender à-go-go: Transsexuals and Drag ♦ 159

14 The Son Also Rises: Daddy/Boy Sex ♦ 169

15 Lie Down With Speed Freaks, Get Up
With No Sleep: Drugs and Need ♦ 183

16 Pampered: Diaper Play and
Other Infantilisms ♦ 201

17 Toward a Topography of Desire:
Summing Up, Kind Of ♦ 215

EPILOGUE: But Even So... ♦ 229

"I hope I'm wearing a leather jacket in my 70s.
I see no reason to return to the middle-class
respectability that it has taken me so long to shed."
—DEREK JARMAN

"What may have intrigued Foucault most about
fist fucking was the way a specific non-normative sexual
practice could come to provide the origin and basis for
such seemingly remote and unrelated events as bake
sales, community fund-raisers, and block parties."
—DAVID M. HALPERIN, *SAINT FOUCAULT*

"Don't dream it, be it."
—*THE ROCKY HORROR PICTURE SHOW*

So what follows, if it's anything classifiable, probably is a travelogue. I've arranged things loosely by topic rather than chronologically. In the cum-soaked pages that follow, I'm going to revisit some of the places I've been and try to make a little more sense of it all. I'll be stopping at a bunch of delightfully squirmy spots, telling some dirty stories, and pondering What It All Means. I'd be pleased if you'd come along. If you've never been to these neighborhoods, I hope you find the vicarious journey one worth taking. And if you have traveled through Kinkland, or if you already make one perverted village or dank-but-inviting valley your home, I hope you find my reflections on the scene to be insightful, amusing. Or maybe so damn maddening that you'll want to go back to the places I describe, if only to prove me wrong.

A few notes here.

Everything in this book is true. More or less. I've changed names and enough details to allow for a degree of plausible deniability, and since I wasn't taking notes in bed, some of the details are…er…well, let's just say the old memory's not what it used to be. But I've tried my best not to lie. Honest.

Also, please believe me when I say that I'm not trying to denigrate any of the topics in this book by bringing it under the "kink" umbrella. I'm sure that some transsexuals will be offended by being grouped with foot fetishists, and vice versa. No offense intended; I respect you all. And I love a lot of you. Especially when you're naked.

One final, important thing before we push off into darkest Kinkland. I'm in a wonderful long-term relationship. It's totally open, loving, and supportive. Without my partner, my wanderings down the primrose paths to Hell would have been a lot riskier, emotionwise. After a hard night sailing down the

Amazon of lust, it's good to have a warm pair of arms to come home to. My partner's taught me a lot (including how to cruise public rest rooms), and I adore him. I believe in love and I believe in commitment. He is, however, largely absent from these pages. That's the way he wanted it and, after all he's put up with, honoring his wishes is the least I can do in return.

OK, guys, cock rings and poppers packed? Then let's hit the road…

I Like to Do *That?*

Last night I flogged my bottomboy again.

Every whack brought a squirm of pleasure. His dick was rock-hard. I was having a great, sadistic time. But while part of my engorged brain watched myself bringing the flogger down upon his tender shoulders, I had to wonder, as I've often wondered, *How did I get here?* How did a nice Jewish boy, a boy who wanted to grow up to be a pharmacist (or, in my more ambitious moments, a rabbi) wind up being a pornographer with a tied-up young masochist in his bed? Well, sure, *everybody's* life is a long, strange trip, but this particular hell-bound trajectory may be a bit, well, *stranger* than most. It's been an odd little odyssey, me afloat on a whirling confluence of gay liberation, the zeitgeist, spiritual seeking, good old-fashioned perversion, and more than a little plain old lust. My Mom would be appalled. G-d would be appalled. Hell, even the Buddha would probably be appalled. And sometimes…sometimes I myself…ah, but the flogger came down again and again while my dick stayed hard. Really hard.

Listen, I'm far from the best top in town. My bondage skills, once finely honed, have grown a bit rusty. My toy bag reflects a freelance writer's income; it's pretty lightweight. And sometimes, when I see a studded leather sash proclaiming the wearer Mr. Leather So-and-so of Two-thousand-something, I have to stifle a giggle. An unlikely hybrid of the Marquis de Sade and Candide, I blunder through the Wonderful World of Sexual Weirdness with my eyes half shut and fingers crossed, hoping for the best. And in that respect, dear reader, perhaps I'm a lot like you.

In fact, as these things go, I came rather late to the party. Way back before HIV and gentrification hit San Francisco like a double whammy, I wandered through 1970s leather bars like a clueless pup. Making my way from the Arena to Folsom Prison to Black and Blue, I'd gape at the whips and chains, then settle for the weak beer of a blow job in the back room. Sure, the sado-maso signifiers were there for any fool to see—hell, I used to attend "slave auctions" where naked guys were "sold off" to the highest bidder. But if anyone had suggested I go home with Mr. Master and spend the evening in handcuffs and pain, I would have either stared mutely or run the other way. Or maybe stared mutely and *then* run.

So, yeah, sometimes I figure I'm the only San Franciscan fag of a certain age who *didn't* fist guys at the Catacombs or the Slot, *didn't* piss on guys at the Caldron. What a pussy I was!

Back then I was so thoroughly clueless that when I thought of sadomasochism at all, I envisioned a slavering monster with a whip, running around trying to find someone slow-moving enough to be forced to give in to his monstrous desires. Little did I suspect that the world was full of hungry bottoms looking for a top skilled enough, caring enough, kinky enough, and willing enough to give them what they needed. Yes, those were innocent days, those times of "Old Guard" leathermen and an underground sexuality that hadn't yet been splashed across music videos, glossy fashion spreads, and a plethora of how-to books for sale at your local Books-A-Million. Oh, the dear, dead days before Madonna—what carefree times they were!

I can easily recall how I finally lost my S/M cherry. I was at Collingwood Park, a late-night cruising ground on the edge of the Castro District. I was making out with a attractive guy with a hard-on, and things were becoming increasingly intense, even a tad kinky. Like any good top-in-training, I was following his every cue, even if I only dimly understood what was up. I had his hands pinned over his head, up against the chain-link fence, when he said it: "I bet you can be a really nasty top."

"Yes, I can," I found myself saying, in my most convincingly (I hoped) butch tone. *Huh?* I thought. *I can? Well…um…maybe…*

The middle of the sidewalk was hardly the place to prove my toppishness, so we made a date. The next morning I went into research mode. Maybe back then I'd already discovered that thumbed-through copy of *The Leatherman's Handbook* at the Salvation Army. Maybe I'd read a few sick stories in a tattered old copy of *Drummer* magazine. But that was it. I had no real notion of how to proceed.

I did know that my friend Jeane was into S/M, and she knew some guys in the 15 Association, which was, I'd heard, San Francisco's elite corps of leathermen with whips.

"Jeane, Jeane," I implored her like a nervous bride, "whatever am I going to do?"

She gave me the best advice possible under the circumstances. "Calm down," she said, all motherly. "Think about what you really want to do to this guy. Do you want to spank him, tie him up, what? Pick one or two things and do them as well as you can. Remember, you're the top. You're supposed to be in control." (The operative phrase being "supposed to be.")

So I rehearsed my lines, trotted off to Ace Hardware to buy some rope, and, dressed all in black, showed up at the guy's house at the appointed time.

There have been quite a number of bottomboys under the bridge since then (and more than a few tops as well), so it's not all that surprising I don't remember the first one's face. Oddly, though, I do recall the way his room looked—it had plywood paneling on the walls, like a mobile home, and a portable fan in the corner. And I remember just how I tied him up, spewed verbal abuse at him, acted pushy and cocky, and slapped him around.

I was lousy.

But something opened up back then, a window onto my possibilities. It was the first time I acted perfectly nasty during sex, but far from the last.

That was well over a decade and a half ago. I did manage to catch the kink wave before it crested, before every suburb had a shop selling bondage cuffs and paddles, before all the mall rats got their dicks pierced. Yes, Junior, times have changed. But even now, when true transgression is increasingly hard to find, the journey into the darker side of sex is one that each one of us kinksters ultimately has to take for himself. And, consciously done, it can be fulfilling and scary and disgusting. And absolutely, absolutely wonderful. Breathtakingly wonderful. Cosmically wonderful. Oh-my-God-I-can't-believe-I'm-feeling-this-wonderful wonderful.

Last night I flogged my bottomboy again.

Nik is less than half my age, ferociously cute, with a skinny dancer's body and a touchingly voracious appetite for abuse. He is so close to my idea of the perfect bottomboy that I feel fortunate; he knows that, and that gives him power over me, but that's a whole other issue. Because last night I was taking him to his limits—taking him further, in fact, than he's trusted other men to take him. Giving him all he could stand, till his lovely body tensed and shuddered under the rain of blows, till I could sense he was ready to curse me, to beg me to stop. And then I gave him just a *little bit more*. I was making him moan and squirm in pleasure and pain, and we were wrapped in the state of mind I think of as "the darkness." For that moment there was nothing in the whole fucking universe but me and him and our twisted desires. It was just like sex, only even more complicated. And then he implored me, for the umpteenth time that night, to make him cum, and this time I finally reached down and did, we both did, we came, shooting off within a split second of one another, and then I kissed him on his beautiful lips and that was that.

"Wanna jump in the shower?" he asked when he'd caught his breath, and I did, washing him down, all glossy and wet and for the moment mine. And then we had a cup of tea.

Ah yes, kinky sex. It is, if you want to be medieval about it, an alchemical transformation. If you want to get all Eastern, it's the union of yin and yang. Nietzsche your boy? Then it's beyond good and evil, *übermensch* sex in all its willful glory. Foucault? Resistance to normalizing discourses. And for the rest of us, it's the good, dirty fun you have on a Saturday night.

In any case, it's a trip. And a journey. I'm not, despite what an article in a local sex magazine said, "one of the kinkiest denizens of San Francisco." Hell, I doubt I'm one of the kinkiest denizens of my *block*. I don't think of myself as some sort of super cocksman. Nor an expert on this or that perversion. I'm certainly not the roughest, handsomest, or best top in town. And Jesus knows that my bottoming talents pale beside some of the delightful pussyboys I know.

I'm just some twisted guy who finds himself on a lifelong journey of discovery, weird tours though the erogenous zone, misadventures below the belt.

Like all of us, I'm just a tourist on the highway of life, each of us on his own journey of erotic discovery. Many of us will settle, happily, for absolute vanilla. But a goodly number of us will visit one place or another in the Land of Kink, if only for vacation, a *tour de perv.* Some of us will doggy-paddle near the shore of Lust Lake, while others will swim right out to the deeps, getting a lot more twisted than I'd dare. There's no right way, there's no single map. For better or worse—for better *and* worse—we make up our lives as we go along.

CHAPTER 1
Satori in the Men's Room: Glory Holes and Bathroom Sex

It started, as many another weird adventure has started, online. I was invited over to a guy's house to stick my cock through his homemade glory hole and get sucked off. OK, sure, why not?

He's left his front door open, as promised, and when I walk into the apartment, somebody else is already there. A somebody pressed up against a door, his pants down around his ankles, his hairy butt cheeks clenched. As I watch, the stranger pumps into the presumed (though unseen) hole in the door, faster and faster, grabbing at the wall for support, until he groans, sighs, and halts his door-fucking. He steps away and pulls up his pants. I never even get to see his dick. Discreet.

My turn. There's an irregularly shaped hole chopped into the center of the wooden door. Not a very professional job, really, and a washcloth or two has been laid on the edge, protection from splinters. On the other side of the hole is a mouth, just that. An open, waiting mouth. I want to see more, but when I ask, the mouth mutters, "We agreed this would be the scene. Give me your dick."

So I do. From what I can see through the glory hole, he's an attractive man, the kind of guy I'd want to approach in a bar. But that isn't the point. The point is that I'm a dick, he's a mouth, and that's all there is to that. Maybe it confirms the dark mutterings of the religious right. Maybe it justifies the condem-nations of old-fashioned shrinks. But at the moment, he and I aren't fully rounded people with complex emotional lives. He's a mouth. I'm a hard-on. Your mother would be appalled. Fuck your mother.

Fuck everything but him swallowing down my hard flesh, coaxing jism out of my balls, up into my shaft, out of my slit, down his hungry, anonymous, dehumanized throat. Is this any way to live one's life? No. Is this pro-gay, healthy, constructive? No, no, and no. But for a time inside a stranger's apartment, inside a stranger's mouth, using a man who, for no doubt dys-functional reasons of his own, doesn't want me even to see him, none of that matters. None of it.

Long before I knew the difference between a flogger and a bullwhip, I used to have sex in public rest rooms. I don't any more—well, hardly ever—but I can't say I regret my time on the tiles. Tearoom sex, as it's called, is the great democracy of dick.

Samuel R. Delany's terrific book *Times Square Red, Times Square Blue* eulogizes the pre-Disney-and-Giuliani-cleanup heyday of gay porno theaters in Manhattan as a time when classes and races of queer men could meet and mix in that rather fetid meat market of life. If that was true of the Adonis Cinema, it's all the more true of the room marked MEN. Oh sure, there's much to be said against the indiscriminate giving of oneself to horny, hard strangers in sordid, stiff-dick circum-stances that invite discovery and danger. Wait…let me compose myself… There, that's better.

Those of us with elevated ideals may find the very idea of bath-room sex to be dehumanizing, degrading, and just plain wrong. One prevalent theory is that this sort of behavior is a vestige of our oppression. Homophobia leads us to think less of ourselves.

Internalizing society's disapproval, we approach ourselves and other queer men as less than human: just dicks. Sucking dick in a toilet stall, the story goes, furthers our own oppression. And who, no matter how horny, really wants to do that?

Certainly, there's an element of truth to that line of thought. Even more crucially, public sex is oft performed by men who are closeted, unwilling to risk self-exposure to satisfy their hungers; many a wedding ring has sparkled beneath a grimy rest-room partition. (Though of course, the ironic fact is that getting busted at a roadside rest stop is likely to lead to a more destructive sort of exposure than voluntarily coming out ever could. So be careful out there, you cheating sons of bitches.)

Quite apart from all that, though, some of us, even us mucho liberated, publicly queer men, just plain *like* fleeting, anonymous encounters. Tsk, tsk, tsk.

Flesh. That's what we're made of. That's what we are. Maybe this anonymous sort of thing is sacred. Maybe it's sick. Maybe it's a bit of both. But I know that, for all the support my primary relationship offers, for all the fun I've had with fuck buddies, as much as I enjoy being with whole people rather than disembodied dicks, there's something about brutally anonymous sex that's special in and of itself. You want fellowship? Go join the Metropolitan Community Church.

There is, I think, something inherently self-annihilating in the human consciousness. I don't know whether it's about the search for nirvana or a marker of mankind's seemingly inevitable slide toward disaster, but whatever it is, there's no use pretending the self-obliterating streak isn't there. And sex gives us the quickest, easiest, safest route to that kind of ego loss celebrated in both the *Tao Te Ching* and *The Story of O*. Eros and Thanatos—it takes two to tango.

The Tibetan Buddhists, it's said, require initiates to spend a night sleeping with corpses. Understanding the transitory nature of all things...isn't that what enlightenment's all about? So what's so weird about finding satori in a men's room?

E-e-ewww, the more fastidious among you might think. And yes, that repulsion is part of the fun, I think. Whatever created us placed, in its wisdom, the organs of excretion and reproduction right next door to one another. For all the trimmings of romance, it's a fact: The pleasures of the asshole go both ways. Piss and cum both flow from the same fount. And bathroom sex is the shrine of those (not necessarily) uncomfortable truths. You sit there, reading half-scrubbed-off graffiti, waiting for a kindred soul to find his way into the next stall as men shit and piss around you, and then the foot appears beneath the partition, tapping, your foot moves in response, and you have a hard-on, yes you do, and the sounds and smells of excretion are part of it, yes they are. Sleeping with corpses.

I remember when I first started cruising men's rooms. I was going to City College, taking art courses. It didn't take me long to discover that the men's room in the Visual Arts building was a nonstop party of sorts. The first boy I ever tricked with there was a perfectly Waspy blonde, clean-cut and irresistible. Every time I saw him, Boy Next Door wore a snowy-white fisherman's knit sweater, the kind his mom would have knitted for him. And when I first risked it, sucking him off beneath the partition, then slipping into his cubicle and sucking his cock while he sat on the toilet, it was a revelation of sorts.

My career at City College was thereafter filled with impromptu orgies during class breaks, and I spent hours after my last class sprawled in a *schmutzy* sort of ecstasy. Men with pale lines where their wedding bands had been, young cholos with earnest uncut dicks, a football player with his foot in an unforgettable cast, prissy queens who sprayed cologne on their crotches (and wasn't *that* an evil idea?). It was in that rest room that I learned of the startling malleability of desire. Given the right circumstances, I learned, I could have sex with damn near anybody, at least anybody with a dick. And that wasn't a bad thing born of insufficient self-respect and tawdry desperation. No, it was a gift.

Times changed. The college administration wised up. How could they not? The blue-painted metal partitions in that rest room had sprouted holes the size of Yosemite Valley—makeshift doorways to grace surrounded by jottings telling of assignations sought and kept, and crude but effective drawings of erections. Every so often the graffiti was erased or overpainted, only to reappear like some persistent case of crabs. Metal plates were bolted over the glory holes. Around the time I finished my time at City College, the doors to the stalls were removed. Paradise lost.

Now, one may argue against tearoom sex on many counts. It is, patently, illegal, and fairly unhygienic as well. The Visual Arts fuckfest undoubtedly made some straight guys—and maybe a few fastidious queers—uncomfortable. There was that telltale rustling of clothes and clanking of belt buckles whenever someone went in to take a piss. Guys shamelessly hung around doing nothing but each other. Horny smokers filled the place with toxic fumes, literate types littered the floor with love notes scrawled on toilet paper. There was a buildup of cum stains on the metal walls. Who knows, some poor soul could have slipped on a recently spurted puddle of jizz and fallen and hurt himself. And there was the specter of HIV, though truth be told, oral sex is pretty far down on the risk continuum, and ass-fucking is rare in the rest rooms. The main course in the tearoom is less likely to get you in viral trouble than what might more easily transpire in some perfectly bourgeois bedroom.

But mostly, the crackdown on roadside sex, sex in the bath-room at the mall, the library, the steam room at the gym, wher-ever the urge to spurt asserts itself, goes back to a simple pro-scription: Sex must be kept tethered. There's a time and place for everything, and boys, *this* ain't the place. I guess it's just that no one's ever answered "Why ain't it?" to my thorough satisfaction.

There are other venereal venues besides the truck stop and the alley, places that in certain jurisdictions are more or less per-missible spaces for anonymous sex. Sex clubs, bathhouses, admission-charged sex parties, adult theaters, video booths, and back-room bars—each is fine in its way. But they still cordon off sex into a zone of separation. More than any other place where large numbers of men have sex with each other, the public rest room makes it thoroughly obvious that there is no impermeable border between our desires and the rest of our lives. Even in the most mundane surroundings love can blossom, if only faceless-ly, if just for a minute or two.

Rest rooms are the only easily accessible public spaces where it's all right to whip out your dick. Once it's out there, its multi-purpose nature becomes clear. *OK, I gotta piss, but while it's here in my hand...* The men's room is where we can let little Willie out, and if he wants to play, who are we to argue? The public bathroom, whether at the local department store, the bus sta-tion, or the roadside rest stop, is where other things come out as well. The good ol' toilet stall (the one with "Tap foot for blow job" written on the wall), where one need only be seen from the waist down, allows even the most straitlaced, closeted man to get off in relative anonymity, though not in perfect safety. For that moment, it's not about who you are, what your job is, what you think and feel and believe. It's about your dick, and your dick can lead you into all sorts of places, both nice and not-so. Small wonder that the cock-size holes chopped through toilet partitions are known as "glory holes." Not only does the term have heavenly resonances, it's also an old-time miners' term. Glory holes are where you go down, deep underground, to find and bring up treasure.

But, like mining for gold, cruising tearooms is not without its dangers. You risk robbery, violence, disease, and perhaps most perniciously, the aforementioned threat of exposure and arrest. The police, in their wisdom, have spent untold dollars and man-hours in pursuing the victimless crime of anonymous cock suck-ing, and as a result, more than one career has gone, more or less literally, down the toilet. Singer George Michael, busted for "lewd conduct" in 1998, said, "My life hadn't been about me forever. And suddenly, it was a way of making my life about me. And for six months, it worked."

Then, too, there's always convenience. Glory-hole sex is the fast-food franchise of lust. Are you in a strange city, looking to get off? Most any hour of the day or night, an all-male theater or dirty bookstore awaits you just down the block. Wanna spurt? Just stick your dick through that hole there. That's it, stick it through.

Forbidden sex is one of the more rankling issues for the queer community at large. Respectable Gay Leaders, the ones who fight for our right to join the army and wed, are hardly eager to fight police surveillance of that toilet out on the interstate. And I can see why. In my nightmares, some member of the Christian right will get hold of this book and read sections of it into the Congressional Record as proof positive of how depraved we all are.

I remember the moment at the first queer March on Washington when I was handed the inaugural issue of *Steam* magazine. *Steam,* the brainchild of the late Scott O'Hara, was chiefly devoted to the nurturance of sex in public places. Lavishly produced in an easy-to-carry format, *Steam* featured articles like "Cruising the Restrooms of Romania" and "Where to Get Rimmed in Montana." Fairly immediately, controversy arose: By publicizing cruising grounds in print, wasn't *Steam* letting cops and bashers know where to attack? These days, when anyone with a computer, from Grandma to the Ku Klux Klan, can go online and find out the same information from tell-all Web sites, the concerns about *Steam* seem almost quaint. (One thing the Web sites don't feature, however, is O'Hara's marvelously literate crusade to sanctify slutdom.)

Meanwhile, no matter what Respectable Gay Leaders say, regardless of the danger, despite the somewhat degrading surroundings (and maybe *because* of all three), it's a safe bet that public sex in non-sanctioned spaces will endure. Be it ever so antisocial, there's just something about it that's irreducibly hot.

As I matured into a well-rounded slut, I began to frequent some of the sex spots that didn't feature plumbing. There were back-room gay bars, the drink-and-suck emporia which flourished in pre-AIDS San Francisco. Though sometimes the orgy rooms were indeed in "back," you could walk into the notorious Boot Camp bar and get fucked right there in the front room, in full view of the bartender. It was all very al fresco but not quite impromptu; you had to plan to go to the bar, knowing full well you'd be trying to score.

Less contrived if more perilous were the assignations in parks or on the beach. Out on the cliffs by the Pacific, there was no telling what you'd find. One sunny afternoon, the prize was a hunky man, shirtless, all muscles and freckles, walking his golden retriever. With a silent Thank You to the Goddess of Cruising, I caught his eye. Within minutes we were safely ensconced in a little clump of trees, and Fido was chained up nearby, just far enough from us to keep his nose out of things. The All-American boy, shorts around his ankles, was sprawled over a log. As the ever-so-scenic waves crashed below us, I fucked his ass. A couple of other cruisers wandered by. One pulled out his own cock and started wanking, circumspectly joining the seaside party. I came, dog-walker came, the voyeur came, we cleaned up as best we could, and we went on our ways. Innocent. Perfect. Ecological. And, decades later, I can still recall how his hard-on looked.

Nothing perfect lasts forever, of course, and within a few years of that shoreline idyll, San Francisco had changed. Four little letters brought the orgy to a screeching halt. In the midst of untold viral misery and death, the back-room bars cleaned up their act or were shuttered, the city put the gay bathhouses out of business, and the parks started a policy of defoliation not seen since the Vietnam War. Outdoor cruising grounds that had been bosky dells of dick sucking were now patrolled by cops on dirt bikes. Medicine met morality, and lust was the loser.

All that's not to say that even hard-core sex hounds shouldn't have some regard for keeping public spaces user-friendly for all comers. I remember one afternoon in an ocean-view trysting spot when I came across two attractive men in a good-size clearing, one leaning against a tree, the other on his knees, giving head. As I stood watching, getting hard myself, a yuppie couple, man and woman, in full jogging gear came trotting through the clearing, just yards away from the blow job. The cocksucker gave them a sidelong glance but didn't miss a beat. Neither sweaty joggers nor shameless boys were fazed, the moment passed, and life, full and bountiful, went on.

I was nearly done writing this chapter when I took a break and went to the movies at a funky but chic theater that shows foreign films. Just before the feature started, I went to take a leak. A cute, slightly heavy man in his late 30s was washing his hands as I stood at the urinal, trying to ignore him long enough to piss. He looked at me and smiled, and I'm quite sure I smiled back. Eventually I gave up and made some inane remark about the turquoise-blue water in the bowl. In less than a minute we were holding hands. He guided my hand to his crotch. He was hard. As was I. My brand-new boyfriend walked to a urinal and pulled out his cock. Pretty! I stroked it for a moment. "We should get back to the theater," he said. "I'm with a…friend."

"OK," I replied, "but would you give me your phone number?"

He did, we made a date, and what happened in the men's room was more fun than the film. In a world where delayed gratifications and sublimated lusts are the rule, the dick rampant had triumphed again.

Yes, men are pigs, and freed from the "civilizing" restraints of women, male-male sex can be even piggier. And yes, many a man, even the straightest arrow, the most pious Christian, the most majoritarian moralist, will let his cock get sucked by a faceless stranger if the moment's right. This is, say most people publicly, a Bad Thing. No, argues a band of sexual liberationists, it's actually a Good Thing. Well, whatever. It's a Thing, and not all the undercover cops in Utah will close it down anytime soon. The yen for sexual pleasure, erotic ecstasy, is so hardwired into most of us that any excuse for a blow job seems plausible in a pinch.

As if an excuse were needed.

CHAPTER 2

Just Looking, Thanks: Exhibitionism, Voyeurism, and Three-Ways

AOL again. The world of online cruising has transformed the sex hunt for many of us, for no matter how denigrated, Net-shopping for nookie does have its pluses. Even if everyone on AOL but me has at least a nine-inch cock. For one thing, it de-emphasizes the visual. There's the attention-getting screen name, the intriguing profile, and only then, usually, do visual specifics come into play. Desire has become a lot more abstract.

Anyway, it's past 2 A.M., I'm horny, he's horny, and we're both online. Do I want to go by his place, stand on the front porch and look through his window, and watch him jack off?

Um, sure.

It seems a bit risky, OK, but I know the neighborhood. Not much chance of being picked up by the cops, I'm hoping.

I park in front of his house—anyway, the address he gave me—a single-family cottage on a quiet little street. Pathway to the front door. Small porch, as described, half hidden from street. Picture window. Light on. So maybe this is on the level. Or maybe I'm gonna get busted. As I walk up the darkened path, my cock is hard. Already.

I've actually never done this before. Well, yeah, a long time ago I had a roommate who brought home a trick and I watched them fucking through a corner window without their ever knowing. I came before they did. And since then there's been all the looking around in locker rooms, sex clubs, and the like. And the odd peek through the odd uncurtained window. Binoculars aimed across the street, sure. But never before a full-fledged voyeurism date, where it was agreed we'd never be in the same room, much less touch.

He's there. On the other side of the window, lying back on the sofa, naked, stretched out, arranged so his face can't be seen. But the rest of him is visible, and it is beautiful—ripped abs, nice chest, hairy legs. Best of all, he's playing with his firm, pretty dick. I reach into my pants and stroke away too. I'm reluctant to whip it out, even with my back to the street, but I'm sure as hell not going to leave, not while my very own private sex show is going on.

What is it about voyeurism (and its mirror-image sibling, exhibitionism) that can make them hotter than some "real" sex can be? I was talking to my fuck buddy Juan about it.

"I really don't like going to sex parties and just watching," he said. "I already get kind of shy in that sort of situation, and I don't want to feel like I'm a total wallflower."

"Sure," I said. "That's one way of looking at it, the voyeur as pitiable loser. But there's another way to look at it too. When you're a voyeur, you're being entertained, you're getting off, and you don't have to actually *do* anything but look. All that fun, no work."

There is, of course, an aspect of voyeurism that smacks of theft, like shoplifting sex. Being a Peeping Tom is against the law, and as a nonconsensual invasion of privacy, it jolly well should be. I'm glad I never got caught. But even in more congenial surroundings, such as sex clubs or back-room bars, standing around watching other men have sex can seem predatory and pitiful at the same time. If the object of a voyeur's gaze is a "victim," he's a victim whose desirability holds the viewer in thrall. (I'm not talking about jacking off to a video or watching strippers put on a show. That's a different kind of power dynamic, one mediated by money. I'm speaking here of the very real pleasure of beholding beauty, especially when it has a hard dick.)

The common view of voyeurs as both dangerous outlaws and pitiable wankers recalls homophobic portrayals of queers as both pathetic misfits and ravening monsters. Straight men know the power of the gaze. It's their birthright when it comes to women, but when they themselves are the object of a lustful stare, many of them are a lot less comfortable. Arguments against gays in the military usually fall back on the staring–in–the–shower room scenario. Real men don't fear rape, but they're apparently scared stiff of a lustful glance at their dicks. E-e-ek! Who could enjoy *that*?

Well, exhibitionists could. They understand the power that being desired can bestow. Within a relationship or an arranged scene, showing off can be a flaunting of one's own sexuality, affirmation that, damn, yes I am a sexy piece and deserve to be desired. But harder-core exhibitionism, getting off by showing off to strangers, brings up issues of consent and assault. Flashers? There are plenty of places in this world of ours where public nudity is less of a deal than it is in our post-Puritan society. And I'm considerably less offended by the unexpected sight of a stranger choking his chicken than I am by TV commercials that use punk rock to sell luxury cars. So I think it's kind of sad that exposing one's dickie to a random stranger or two should be construed as sexual assault rather than just bad manners. But then, if it weren't forbidden, exhibitionism wouldn't carry quite the same charge, now, would it?

I can remember poring over nudist camp magazines when I was a kid. (This was in the dim, dead days when gay porn magazines couldn't show cock, but "naturist journals" could.) The save-your-ass pretext was that looking at magazines with photos of blurry-dicked men playing volleyball had everything to do with "the beauty of the human body" but nothing at all to do with eroticism. That was pretty damn disingenuous, though I'd think it probable that in cultures where nudity's more normal—including the Sunnyland Naturist Park—the whole voyeur/exhibitionist thing loses its edge. But back here in repressionland, both looking with lust and sexual showing are still taboo, more or less. (It would be nice to do an anthropological study of cross-cultural kink, so if anyone's handing out grants...)

There *are* semi-sanctioned places where one can be a voyeur and/or exhibitionist without fearing the long arm of the law, but almost all of those, in this charmingly late-capitalist society, are pay-to-get-in spaces. Back in the early days of the epidemic I used to hang out at "Jacks Parties," where 100 or so naked, horny homos crowded into a big warehouse-type room. There were men of varying shapes, sizes, races, ages, with hard-ons of varying sizes and shapes. At Jacks, we all stripped down and did nothing more risky than jerk one other off. Some guys didn't even do that; much of the masturbation was mutual, but some men were in full look-but-don't-touch mode. I clearly recall one buff bruiser, all perfect muscles and beautiful big cock, who stood in a corner all night beating his meat and rebuffing everyone's advances. At the time I had one of those "Who does she think *she* is?" reactions. Stuck up. Thinks he's too good for us. Or else: uptight, his psyche as armored as his body appears to be. I was being, I'll now admit, pretty ungenerous (and maybe a little envious). He was hot. Hot hot hot. I can still vividly (though no doubt inaccurately) remember how his well-formed pecs flexed with every stroke, how he brought his oozing stiffy to the brink of orgasm again and again and again. Fact is, I recall Mr. Untouchable better than anyone I actually played around with at those parties. (Well, with the exception of a local theatrical luminary I subsequently jacked off in Row O of the Castro Theatre during the Queer Film Festival.) Mr. Untouchable was hunky, showed it off, got us off, and got off doing it. So where was the harm? Maybe he wasn't an armored snob at all. Maybe he was just an exhibitionist.

The Jacks was one of the places I learned about the power of the gaze, and the distinction between "a hot guy" and "a hot sexual situation." There's something to be said, of course, for spotting a man, thinking he's the most gorgeous specimen on the face of the earth, approaching him (or maybe better yet, having him approach you), and winding up in bed—or wherever—with him. But just being the object of desire—or conversely, coming on to someone you *know* isn't as hot as you are—can also be powerfully sexy. It's that—the power of desire, the inequalities and mysteries of sexual attraction—that make voyeurism and exhibitionism a lot more complex and interesting than they might seem at, well, first glance.

Listen, I'm not exactly porn-star material, so if a guy plunks himself down next to me in the steam room at the Y and makes his interest known, I pop an immediate stiffy. It's not necessarily the prospect of getting into his nonexistent pants. I can find my admirer to be utterly unattractive and still get off on being stared at. If a cat can look at a king, a troll is welcome to cruise my cock.

I confess, oh yes, I confess… Recently at the gym, I was followed into the steam room by a homely guy with a big ungainly belly. I'm not being snotty here: Brad Pitt I ain't, and I strongly suspect that to some tricks I've been a mercy fuck. I can live with that. But take my word for it, if there were some objective scale of attractiveness, my steam-room stalker would have occupied a lower rung than I. And yet, when he sat very close to me and stared, very obviously, at my cock, said organ began to swell up like nobody's business. When the fellow slid his hand over to my naked, hairy thigh, I not only let him, I enjoyed it. Hell, I not only enjoyed it, I leaned back and thrust my crotch in the air, the better to show off my cock. We didn't really *do* anything. He reached for my dick and squeezed it for a second. I reached down, gave his hand an affectionate squeeze back, and removed it from my erection. I wasn't, after all, about to imperil my membership for the sake of a grope. And back outside in the showers, I acknowledged my suitor's glance but didn't encourage further contact, gratified though I was that he never took his eyes off me.

Was I a coldhearted cocktease? Well, I'd prefer to think I was a site of desire, for those few minutes somebody's sex object. I let him look, I let him touch. I didn't feel violated. I felt empowered.

I once read an essay on steam-room sex by an author who, obviously finding himself a dreamboat, excoriated the ugly old trolls who had the temerity to cruise him. How *dare* they? But their stares weren't an insult to his attractiveness—quite the opposite. Being desired ennobles, not demeans. That whole fag pecking-order thing is so tiresome for those of us not in the top ranks of hunkitude, and even some real beauties have complained to me about the superficiality of it all. Voyeurism is egalitarianism in action, so get over yourself, darling.

It's not only looking that can be sexy. *Not* seeing can be hot too; being deprived of sight can be both disempowering and liberating. I've left blindfolds and hoods outside the door for more than one "blind date," and there have been times when whoever and I played for hours and never saw each other's face. Just last month, there was the husky blond guy who'd left his front door open and awaited me, naked and blindfolded, in his bed. His never seeing my face, only getting to know me by touch, made the afternoon even sexier, more intimate, as though my very anonymity brought us closer. I could have been anyone, everyone. And I was.

And then there was a memorable time that I surrendered *my* sight, and careened toward the edge of safety, to boot.

I'd made contact with the guy on the phone sex lines. He invited me to his house out in the burbs. I was to let myself in, strip, put on a blindfold, and clasp my hands behind my back. Stupid? I was in the mood for adventure, and I figured I could take care of myself. The house was nondescript, middle-class, and the only sound that weekday afternoon was the roar of a distant leaf blower. I went to the door, hoping someone wasn't playing games that would result in my head being blown off by an irate widow with a shotgun. I unlocked the door. So far, so good. I let myself in, stripped, and put on the blindfold that hung from the knob. A door creaked open, then I heard footsteps. My unseen host bound my hands, forced me to my feet, and slapped me hard. A sane man would not have gotten himself into this position. But I was in "this position," and my cock was so hard it hurt.

My unknown master wasn't, truth be told, a very good top, but the situation overrode the details. He was a beefy guy. I could tell from subtle physical clues, like his fat belly pressing into my back. I just hoped he wouldn't try to fuck me without a condom. Turned out I didn't have to worry about that. He'd hardly started in on me when there was a knock on the door. My unseen host half-dragged me across the house and threw me onto a bed, tossing my clothes on top of me. Then he said it: "Stay there and don't move a muscle. You make a noise, and I'll kill you." And he shut the door.

There was a decent possibility that I was playing house with a psychotic murderer. But at least he was a lousy bondage top, for which I was cosmically grateful: It was a cinch to wriggle free of the ropes. I pulled the blindfold off. Yep, the underpants scattered around the floor were big, size 44s. I could still hear voices through the door. Was this a set-up scene, something to frighten the trick? If it was, it was singularly convincing. I wasn't about to take any chances. I threw my clothes on, then lay down on the bed, my back to the door. After a few minutes, the bedroom door opened. "Don't fucking look at me," said a strangled voice. "Get the fuck out, and don't look. I'm warning you."

Well, I didn't need to be told twice. I got the hell out of there, and as I motorcycled down the freeway, I repeated to myself, like a mantra, "Safe sane consensual safe sane consensual…"

The intricate equilibrium of attractiveness and need is daunting enough to have kept me cautious about three-ways. My first ongoing triad involved me, a hairy hunk, and his chubby boyfriend, who liked having two dicks up his ass at once. (I was a *lot* more limber then.) It didn't take me long to realize I was considerably more turned-on by the one with fur than the one with the belly. I was, in fact, only going over to their place and fucking the bottom so my dick could be next to his boyfriend's. By the same token, I'm not sure how either of them felt about me. Maybe the bottom wanted me more than his partner. Maybe not.

And thusly I learned the obvious: When there are three instead of two, one guy is liable to end up odd man out. At least if a one-on-one goes awry, you don't have to lie there rejected and watch two other homos having fun. So it was with some trepidation that a few weeks ago I arranged my first three-way in years. I'd been waiting for Nik to come over and was just killing time on AOL when I ran across Charlie, a boy Nik's age whom I'd played with once before. Unlike Nik, he was more top than bottom (though the first time we met I'd spanked his pretty ass). When I typed to Charlie that I was about to top my favorite masochist, his virtual ears perked up. Could he come over and watch me abuse Nik? And maybe join in? Well, um, sure, as long as it was OK with Nik. But Nik was on his way, and as he doesn't own a cell phone, much less a computer, there was no way to check with him. So I just assumed that he, along with most every bottom I've ever known, harbored a desire to service multiple tops. I invited Charlie over.

Nik was late—Nik is *always* late—so Charlie arrived first. By the time my bottomboy turned up, Charlie had spanked me, flogged me, and permitted me to take off his Nikes and service two of the most attractive feet I'd laid eyes on in quite a while. I'd had no hesitation. Charlie was an attractive young man (and a professional masseur), and if he enjoyed standing there stroking his nipples and paddling my ass, it was no blow to my pride. What it did do was give me a hard-on, so when I went to answer Nik's tardy doorbell ring, my pants were nicely tented out.

"Hey, what's happening?" cute little Nik said, his customary greeting.

"Hi, Nik. I have a little surprise for you."

"Is it a good surprise or a bad surprise?" (I'd inadvertently given him scabies once, so he had reason to be a bit wary. On the other hand, his infected throat had once exposed me to gonorrhea, so I guess it was a wash.)

"A good surprise, I hope." I smiled and led him into the living room, where Charlie sat, beautifully barefoot, seeming a bit distant, but both hands under his sweatshirt, playing with his tits.

We all agreed that the surprises were good. Nik pulled down my pants and started sucking my cock. Charlie sat there watching, hands still on his nipples, not going to the dick that was now visibly swollen inside his shorts. Nik and I were onstage, and the boy who'd been my top just minutes before was now the audience, looking on as I was pleasured by a boy whom Charlie quite obviously desired.

Within minutes the three of us were in the bedroom, Charlie perched on a stool, spectatorship intact, watching me and Nik go at it. His voyeurism was both exclusion and privilege, but nobody seemed to mind. Finally, though, I looked in Charlie's eyes, then down at his bulging basket, and said to Nik, "Go suck his cock." Nik peeled off Charlie's shorts, revealing a really nice, really stiff dick, and serviced Charlie as I watched, the voyeur position now mine. For the next hour or two, things constantly shifted between us. The new boy was the object of Nik's and my attentions, Nik sucking his dick while I ate his ass. Then I sat watching as Nik and Charlie "performed" for me, Nik sucking cock while getting spanked. I was left out as the two young guys played, but I was also in supreme control—it was my bed, and I'd arranged the party. Two cute boys doing each other just inches away? I was in provisional heaven. Then I joined in again, spanking Charlie and getting swatted in turn as Nik, watching us, stroked his dripping dick. Eventually, things centered on me and Nik: me slapping, spanking, and finally fucking his tight ass while Charlie watched. And then, when none of us could wait much longer, the three of us shot our wads in perfect porn-video synchronization, me filling the condom up Nik's ass, Nik sperming all over himself, and Charlie spraying spunk over us both. Bingo!

After Charlie had left, Nik and I talked in the shower.

"I think that went really well," I said, soaping Nik's asshole. "We all kept things balanced."

"Yeah," said Nik. "I did my best. But I think things were a maybe a little strange because the two of us—"

"Are 27 years old?" I impulsively blurted out.

"No," said Nik, "I meant you and me. We were so obviously into each other that I hope Charlie didn't feel left out."

Which just goes to show you: "Who's the mercy fuck?" is a matter of opinion, and there's nothing like a three-way to keep the ambiguities flying.

Then, just the other day, I'm taking a break from work when I make online contact with a 30ish Asian-American with a hungry ass. We swap pics. Do I want, he asks, to come over and fuck him?

"Only if I can eat it first," I haggle. I'm shrewd.

We talk by phone to set things up. "Do you mind," he asks, "if a friend comes over and watches you fuck me?"

I've been working on the voyeurism chapter; how can I object? More research. More research.

An hour later I'm climbing his front stairs. Turns out the picture he's sent me was, well, flattering. But he's still fuckable. As we enter his living room, he gestures toward another young man. "This is my friend Vito." Vito extends a hand. He's yummy, just short of handsome, a little rough around the edges. He can watch me any time.

"Let's head up to the bedroom."

Ken and I are in bed and Vito's leaning in a corner when I say it: "I think you should get closer, Vito. Real close, so you can see."

Vito has his really nice dick in his hand as I lick Ken's ass and suck his dick. God, Vito's a hunk. Then *he* says it, to Ken: "You want me to fuck you?"

"Yeah," says Ken. "You want to?"

Hey! Just a dang minute here! What about me?

But Vito is already pulling a condom on his fine Italian cock. Ken's ass is kind of tight, but soon enough he's getting pumped vigorously, doggy-style, as I watch, hard dick in hand.

"You want to get under him?" Vito asks. Or commands.

"And do what?"

"Maybe suck his cock."

Well, it's not an unpleasant prospect, especially since Ken's dick has one of those extra-long foreskins I've lately come to love. But in the event, every thrust of Vito's dick brings Ken's crotch down on me, hard. My face is not only getting fucked, it's getting shmooshed. I arrange myself so that, mouth unoccupied, I can enjoy the close-up view of dick pounding hole mere inches from my face. I might have felt left out, but instead I just feel horny. And perilously close to coming. I restrain myself, scoot around, and plant my tongue up Vito's hairy crack, but that doesn't work too well either; it inhibits his manly Sicilian thrusts. So I eventually just lie there watching.

Vito comes, pulls out, tosses his clothes back on, and leaves.

"So he's a fuck buddy of yours?" I ask when the front door has clicked shut.

"Yeah," Ken says. "I've known him for a while. I think he was a little weirded out. I told him about you and he said he wanted to come over, but...well, I think he felt uncomfortable."

"I couldn't tell."

"Well, I could. Hey, you want to fuck me?"

But my cock, having been restrained from coming, then having been ignored, is now probably too shy to stay stiff in a condom. And I don't really mind.

"Don't think so."

But thanks for asking.

And that guy in the cottage, stroking off behind his window?

Well, we'd agreed it was to be a pure show-off scene, so I stand there watching till I'm convinced every cop in town is at my back. But eventually I can restrain myself no longer. Screw the prearrangements, I knock on the guy's door. He is, fortunately, no stickler; he lets me in. I suck on that nice, juicy dick, and he, in turn, goes down on me. Yes, I can appreciate all the glories of exhibitionism and voyeurism, all that stuff. But I'm afraid that, for me, there's nothing like the feel of a real, hard, hot cock. I guess I'm just not a very good Peeping Tom.

CHAPTER 3

This Little Piggy: Foot Fetishism

OK, feet.

Feet?

I mean, there are perversions and then there are *perversions*. On the one hand, there are nice, respectable kinks like sado-masochism, with its chic leather garments, pricey accoutrements, and tie-ins to MTV. But even in these kink-friendly times, it's easier to boast about branding a guy and shitting in his mouth while listening to *Turandot* than it is to confess that sucking on a guy's attractive toes makes your dick hard.

Sucking on a guy's attractive toes makes my dick hard.

There, I've said it and I'm not ashamed. Much.

"My name is Simon and I like feet."

"Hello, Simon."

Talk about your 12-step programs...

Does footlove make sense? Nope. But it's precisely the inexplicable, nonfunctional, nearly antifunctional nature of foot fetishism that charms the pants off me. Yeah, I know the Freudian line about the Dick Displaced Downward. And I'm not unaware of the cozily submissive aspects of foot worship. Not to mention all those nerve endings—the foot *is* an erogenous zone, after all. And sure, the grown-up perv no doubt resonates to infantile memories of rug-ratting around Dad's big, powerful loafers. Or if we want to get spiritual about it, there's even ol' J.C. Himself, raptly washing His hunky disciples' tootsies. Then there's astrology: This is, I'm assured, the Piscean Age, and Pisces rules—of course—the foot. But, but…

But in an age of numberless how-to-be-bent books and endless talk-show sex chat, in an era when the daily paper—at least in San Francisco—carries Tips on Anal Sex, I long (as you might have gathered by now) for the return of mystery. Good sex should be a what-the-fuck-was-*that*? And feet, or rather, what's hot about feet, can never quite be fully explained away. When the socks come off, the dick goes up. What more does one need to know?

My way kinky leatherdyke pal Robin says to me, "I can't understand foot worship. *Boot* worship, sure…" What can I reply? "Screw you and your vanilla tastes"?

Indeed, any fetish worth its salt is pretty much a cosmic mystery, though the less charitable might term it a cosmic joke. The eroticization of something that's not directly sexual, or focusing all one's sexual energy on, say, the ball sac or the nipple, is, to those not in on the fetish, pretty weird. I can understand, for instance, leather fetishes, though I really don't partake. But the wonderful world of rubber is still terra semi-incognito to me. Sure, I can appreciate my friend Marc in his latex cat suit, sleek black rubber hugging every curve, wrapped around his butt, cradling his big dick. But just why some guys get hard at the sight of fisherman's waders or a fireman's yellow rubber coat is, frankly, a bit beyond my ken. I know they're not fibbing about their lusts, so in the spirit of We're All in This Together, I respect their fetishes, no matter how bizarre, arcane, risible. Because, after all, toes make my cock ache.

Which is not to say that foot sex is a simple phenomenon. In an age of specialization, even the kinks have kinks. The late, lamented *Foot Scene* magazine ("Cover-boy Tyler and His Size 14s!") carried classified ads that beggared the imagination of the non-aficionado. Talk about specialized tastes! Jocks in smelly high-tops. Middle-aged black guys in semitransparent dress socks with opaque heels and toes. Adidas only, please. Or tassel loafers with worn-down heels. Fourteen-eyelet versus 10-eyelet lace-up work boots...the debate rages on. Each brand of boot has its own fan club, its own mystique. Even Teva sandals have their fans. Not Nike sandals, which just won't do. *Tevas!* (In late-consumer-capitalist sex, there's nothing like brand loyalty.) Your average Teva worshiper must be in hog heaven whenever summer rolls around. Whilst strolling around town, he probably spends so much time looking downward that he runs smack-dab into light poles and stop signs and stuff. All that pain, just for a glimpse of overpriced nylon webbing, crisscrossing flexing, shining foot flesh. Life is, indeed, rich and strange.

And that brings us to the thing itself: the foot. Stripped of footwear, the male foot stands revealed as an object of desire, a form divine. Bones and tendons, joints and veins, more complex even than a dick. And, like penises, each and every foot has a personality all its own. What infinite variety! Long, elegant toes. Broad, butch little feet. Arches high or not so. Toes hairy or smooth. Clean. Slightly smelly. Reeking. Ah, the rhapsody!

(A little postmodern aside here: Even as I write this, I feel a bit of queasiness at this degree of self-revelation. A trace of shame. As though I'm fucking up my toppish credentials. As though I should be writing about something *butch*, like diaper scenes. But that'll come later...)

Then there's the safe-sex angle. Forget about condoms; socks are all that foot sex requires. Well, sure, there's the possibility of picking up a staph infection or something from wherever those feet have been. Not to mention fungus: A while back I saw an ad on a foot-play Web site placed by a guy who, in all apparent seriousness, was turned on by advanced cases of athlete's foot. Sort of the foot-fetish version of scat play, I guess. *Too heavy a scene for me, bud. Even tops have their limits.* On the other hand, a bit of natural tang doesn't hurt. I don't really want the objects of my affection to smell of nothing more enticing than Irish Spring. The bacterium that causes feet to smell is, after all, pretty much the same microorganism that ripens your finest Brie. Gourmet tastes both.

I used to be on the staff of a gay men's S/M party that met in the downstairs dungeon of a two-story warehouse. The upstairs was rented by the Foot Fraternity. Simultaneous parties. It sure was fun to be the doorman. It was easy to tell where a new arrival belonged just by looking at him from the ankles down. Polished motorcycle boots…downstairs. Suede Airwalks…going up! Downstairs, the party got rolling to the sound of slaps and moans and barked orders, a dungeonful of studied hypermasculinity. But upstairs (and I *did* slip upstairs…don't tell) things were different. Quiet. Peaceful. Guys chowing down on one another's insteps, nothing louder than sniffing and slurping. It was like a Zen garden of perversion, all carefully raked gravel and moist size 10s. And if, on occasion, I slipped off my big black boots and sank into a puppy pile of mutual sock-stroking…well, I'm not ashamed, got that? NOT ASHAMED!

Not that the two worlds can't sometimes meet. I used to have a footslave: a big, handsome, clunkily masculine guy who loved being at my feet. Well, actually, he loved being at *someone's* feet; as is the case with many another kink, a certain instrumentalism was at work, and I sometimes felt that I was just the human being connected, somewhat inconveniently, to the 10 toes of my slaveboy's desires. Still, I did my best, tying him down, taking off my old, extremely stinky leather high-tops and spreading a Reebok sneaker over his face. Slaveboy would lie there, breathing in my stench, as I rubbed my bare feet over his torso, down to his swollen dick. This would go on for hours, but he never seemed to lose interest. Or his erection. Good top that I am, I focused in on his body, his excitement, the eroticism of my power position, and I enjoyed myself quite a lot, eventually jacking off and then putting my shoes back on. If slaveboy had been a very good lad that day, I'd even shoot spooge onto my feet and let him lick them off.

Recently I took a footslave (a different one—the world being full, as we all know, of eager bottoms) to a party at a local dungeon. I got him down on the floor, tied that same old stinky leather high-top over his handsome face, and stood on his chest. Meanwhile, not 10 feet away, a hooded man was chained to a cage, dick mummified in an Ace bandage, while a man in chaps slid needles through his skin. And across the room, a nasty bear used his single-tail whip on a bleeding man bound to a St. Andrew's cross. Those were *real* scenes. And all the leatherguys who saw me feeding my dirty socks to my footslave seemed, well…bemused. In those circumstances, it would have taken guts for me to relinquish my top position and do what I ached to do, which was to kiss my footslave's bare feet, so shapely, so pretty, so big. (No, I'm really not a size queen, but in feet, as in meat, largeness does have a certain appeal.)

Perhaps "relinquish my top position" overstates the case, though. After all, a top is *supposed* to be able to do whatever he damn well pleases. Right? *Right?!?*

And one thing I want to do, what I have in fact on occasion done, is this…

The bottom is tied spread-eagle to the bed, naked except for a hard-on, a blindfold, and a pair of—let's make them thick woolen socks, the gray-with-a-red-stripe kind. (It sort of worries me that the bottom, stripping down at my command, has neglected to take off his socks. Are his feet deformed? Unattractive?

One otherwise-cute playmate turned out to have yellowed toe-nails and weirdly misshapen toes, thus robbing me of a site of desire. But perhaps this one has kept his socks on merely as a striptease of sorts. Or a fashion statement. Or perhaps he's just chilly.) Spread-eagle Boy is nervously anticipating clothespins on his nipples, cock-and-ball torture, a riding crop applied smartly to his inner thighs. Instead, I walk to the foot of the bed, undo an ankle restraint, lift his foot, and pull the woolen sock off.

His foot is beautiful.

And it's *mine*, mine to do with as I wish. My caresses may surprise Spread-eagle Boy, but they'll probably delight him as well. The intense sensations of having his foot played with might be new to him, or he might be an old hand, so to speak, at this. And if he's very ticklish, well, it'll just make things more interesting. I bring his bare foot to my lips and gently lick the bottom of his big toe. I can see his dick throb. Yes! My mouth moves down over his sole, instep, arch, my tongue leaving a damp trail of sensation in its wake. A sometimes-devalued, oft-overlooked part of his body is mine to play with, an object of erotic desire *because I say it is.*

My tongue moves between his toes. He gasps. My fingers brush the sole of his naked foot. He twitches, the ticklish sensation becoming nearly too much to bear. But this won't be a tickle-torture scene. And neither will it be a pain scene, with my hand or leather paddle swacking the sensitive soles of his feet. Not yet, anyway. It's too early for what the Spaniards, in their romantic tongue, call *bastinado*. Right now I'm gently screwing around with his right foot, because I'm the top and that's what I choose to do. And what's Spread-eagle Boy going to say? "This is too kinky, drip hot wax on my dick instead"?

His big toe is in my mouth. I suck on it like it's a penis. Perhaps, if I'm feeling greedy, I stretch my mouth over all five toes. Or chew at his arch, his leathery heel. It's a rare bottomboy who can remain impassive through all this. *OK, you tied-up bastard, squirm for me. I want to see you squirm. This little piggy…*

Somewhere along the line I might use his spit-wet feet to jack myself off. I suppose that if I were a truly devoted foot fetishist, I'd want to shoot my load that way, my dick against a beautiful bottom's beautiful feet, cum gushing over toes, insteps, ankles. And in fact I've done just that, at least once or twice. But usually I move on to other things. And if, while I'm fucking a guy with his legs in the air, I grab his graceful ankles and bury my face in his feet, surely he won't protest. *Wee wee wee, all the way home…*

It's odd how obsessive feet can make a fetishist. Take the Foot Bear, for instance. When I get to his house for our online-negotiated date, he unties my shoes, takes one sniff, and suggests, "Use my own socks instead." I'm probably looking dubious. "Please," he begs. And he reaches into a laundry bag and pulls out a pair of over-the-calf black dress socks I can smell from across the room; they clearly haven't been laundered since the days of Oscar Wilde. Now, over-the-calf socks are about as erotic to me as—well, you choose the disparaging simile—but they clearly are giving Foot Bear a chubby, and at least he doesn't want me to wear garters too. He worshipfully pulls my socks off and then, without a second glance at my bare toes, slips the reeking footwear on my feet. Even for me, the smell is a bit much, but for him, it's Magic Time. He gets those socks in his face, in his mouth, in the submissive depths of his rather perverted soul. "Spit," he says, and I do, right on the filthy socks. He licks off my saliva and begs for more. If he isn't precisely My Type, if he looks a lot less butch and somewhat more bulky than the photos he'd E-mailed me, his lust is an instant, insistent turn-on. And buddy, I just love to facilitate obsession. *Hey, are you hopelessly sick and twisted? Here, let me help you with that.*

Foot Bear has one other bit of dirty laundry to share. He reaches into that sacred laundry bag of his and pulls out the single filthiest jockstrap I've ever, ever seen.

"Put this on," he asks. Well, directs. Demands?

That jockstrap is so stiff it might just as well be made of cardboard painted a ghastly shade of ecru. It's so stiff it scratches on the way up. Pulling it over my private parts is icky, though not icky enough to deflate my erection.

"Now go look at yourself," Foot Bear says, gesturing to a full-length mirror in a corner of the room. I do, and can't help but notice I look faintly ridiculous in my T-shirt, filthy jockstrap, and dress socks. In this sort of situation, one of several responses is called for. You can break down in hysterical laughter at the weird perversion, which is to say, a perversion that isn't *yours*. You can apologize profusely as you take off (in this particular case) the piss-stiff athletic supporter while you explain about having to get to an appointment you've suddenly remembered. Or you can do what I do, which is to come out with some variation or other of the now-classic "Get down on your fucking knees and suck my cock."

As they say in porn magazines, he tongues my bulge through the stretchy, smelly pouch, his dick standing at strict attention below the curve of his hairy belly. Then his mouth goes back to those stiff socks: yummy yummy. He is, in some smelly way, in his very own version of Heaven, and I suddenly picture him rifling through Mommy's dirty-laundry hamper, burying his face in the dirty clothes that stink like Daddy. (There are other possible scenarios too, but the weirdly mixed metaphor of the jockstrap and dress socks make this particular narrative an obvious choice.) So I try the Father gambit: "That's it, son, you just wrap your mouth around Daddy's smelly socks." I've poked just the right spot; he damn near loses control. What a needy child this 30-year-old is! If I were a tad more sentimental, it would make me want to cry, though goodness knows Tough Tops Don't Weep.

In a few minutes I've managed to add my own spunk to the crusted-up funk on the socks. Foot Bear licks the jizz off those socks, then comes explosively all over the floor. He's a nice guy, it's a nice moment, and at last I'm able to take that damned uncomfortable jockstrap off.

Later, I get a thank-you note E-mail that reads, "You indulged me in some pigginess that i really really need and never get to do and you did it beautifully." Aw, shucks.

On the other hand—or, to be more precise, foot—the sight and smell of the male foot can turn me into a mass of way-submissive Jell-O, for real. One man, a German fellow, advertised online for a foot pig to worship his stinking sock-clad feet, and my mouth began to water before I'd finished reading his ad.

When he shows up, he's in a business suit, wearing non-descript black oxford shoes. He's handsome, with salt-and-pepper hair and steely-gray eyes, not really my usual type. Nope, not at all. He's no cringing bottomboy. He is, in fact, my very own Daddy, a nasty man with reeking feet, and I'm on my knees in seconds. I grovel, I snuffle, I pull the laces open with my teeth, pull off the shoes, worship his socked feet, which are, indeed, moistly stinking to high heaven.

Herr Vater turns out to be something of a stern disciplinarian. "You're a bad, bad boy," he growls, and who am I to disagree?

When he starts slapping me around, I know I've hit pervert pay dirt. He's not the most skilled sadist in the world: He doesn't know much about pacing or warm-up, and his script is pretty limited, of the unvarying "You're such a naughty, sick boy. Why do you misbehave? Why do you make me do these things to you?" variety. But that's quite enough for me. I maneuver myself into the bottom space where I need to be and become a contrite, suffering little lad who just loves Daddy so much.

Whack. "I promise I'll be better, Daddy." Whack.

In fact, I realize, as the scene surges on, as he discovers the riding crop hanging on the doorknob and gives me half a dozen barely bearable strokes, that the limitations of his script are a virtue. The repetition, the circularity of the verbal play, are like a mantra in some yoga of humiliation. He gives me the cues but doesn't get bogged down in detail. It's your basic, hypnotic call and response.

"You're a bad boy."

"I'm sorry, Daddy."

"You're a dirty boy."

"I'm so sorry, Sir."

The porno simplicity of the dialogue sets me free to discover my own guilt, regret, shame. I scribble a note in my mental Top's Notebook: "Next time, keep things even simpler for whoever's your bottomboy."

I'm extremely grateful. I can't figure out why such a sexy man would want to make me into his boy, give me the gift of his sweaty, rank feet. He *is* only doing this for my own good. What a generous, loving Daddy!

I am not worthy. I am not worthy of his sweaty, filthy, nauseating feet, which is to say, of his overwhelming love. Guilt. Punishment. Forgiveness. Sin. Damnation. And smelly, smelly socks.

Feet, OK?

When you think about it, it's really no weirder to be turned on by a nice pair of feet than by pencil-eraser nipples, a well-filled scrotum, or a hairy butt. Well, OK, maybe it *is* weirder, but fuck it. Author Patrick Califia once said to me, "I mean, what's the use in being a sexual pioneer if you don't chronicle the whole enchilada? "

OK, feet.

CHAPTER 4

Lending a Hand: Fisting and Other Extreme Sex

"I'd like to try something," he says.

"Sure," I say, ear to phone, wondering what.

"I'll leave the apartment door unlocked. I'll be naked face-down on the bed when you arrive, and you can just walk in and start playing with my butt. Fist me, OK?"

That sounds good to me. It will be only the second time we've met, but we have at least played before, so there won't be compatibility questions. The first time, though, he hadn't asked me to fist-fuck him.

"I'll be there in a half hour," I say. "I'll bring the gloves." And I hang up the phone.

His place is in one of those pricey-but-barren apartment complexes with a pool and a doorman. Elevator, long corridor, apartment door. Unlocked. When I walk into his bedroom, I remember why I'd wanted to play with him again. He isn't exactly my type. In fact, he's the diametrical opposite of slacker boys like Nik. He seems like a bank manager. Blond, blandly handsome, with a slightly flabby body and a big, welcoming ass. It's easy to imagine him wearing a suit, sitting behind a desk and turning down mortgage applications. At the moment, though, he's lying naked facedown, a couple of pillows under his belly, his largish butt invitingly presented for use.

I pull off my pants and pull on a pair of latex gloves. He's told me he'd been playing the night before, had only napped a little.

I took this to mean "did speed." Doesn't matter to me. I take a glob of lube and start massaging it onto his hole. He moans. I look around his bedroom. A couple of nice pieces of furniture. No books, nothing very personal except a few framed photos on his bedside table. And on the wall is a big unframed poster of Audrey Hepburn in *Breakfast at Tiffany's*. You know the one: She's looking gorgeous in Givenchy and shades. I slip three fingers into his rump.

Mr. Banker's ass opens up for me, soft as butter. I look up at Miss Hepburn, unflappable behind her expensive sunglasses. As my fingers prowl around soft, yielding insides, I try to imagine myself as Holly Golightly—a wacky, footloose chick with a yen for men. It doesn't work. I remain, stubbornly, a middle-aged homo with my fingers in a blond guy's butt. I pull out, scrunch my pinky down, and reenter him with four fingers. Stretching him out, rotating my hand, I manage to get my thumb in too, and press forward till I'm in up to my knuckles. And then, slowly, gradually, wetly, my whole hand slides inside.

"Moon River" indeed.

Fisting is something of a specialty act. Guys have to train themselves to get fisted, gradually whipping their sphincters into shape till they can take an entire hand. And tops really should know what they're doing. The deeper the penetration, the trickier the terrain and the more danger of doing real physical harm. Like many advanced sexual subcultures, the fisting scene attracts mostly older guys, men who have had time to work up to major-league perversion.

In an era of erotic specialization, it's not surprising that there's a whole fisting subculture, with Web sites, parties, and how-to manuals. There's definitely a fisting circuit in San Francisco, guys with red hankies who show up at all the right sling parties. For a time they even advertised in a national fisting magazine, *Trust*, which grew from a homemade newsletter into a glossy affair, only to cease publication, collapsing like a well-used asshole.

There's something so unnatural about fisting that it makes things pleasantly surreal. There's the buildup: Devoted fistees douche themselves out to keep things from becoming unsavory. And there's the medical snap of latex gloves, and the liberal applications of lube. Lately the community of handballing (as fist fucking's also called) has discovered a great lube, a mix-it-yourself powder designed for use by farmers and veterinarians, men who work with bulls and pigs. This seems about right. It's the reason so many urban fags are now getting catalogs for farm supplies in the mail.

When, in my innocent youth, I first heard about fisting, my jaw must have dropped, I must have thought, *Oh, that's impossible! Up to the elbow?!* But that was a long time ago. I remember the first time I fist-fucked someone, at a bathhouse back in the '70s, and how amazing it was. But lots of things were amazing back then. At the baths one night, I saw an astonishing scene: a man with his arm stuffed into another guy nearly up to the shoulder. I felt like I was in a Bugs Bunny cartoon, eyes popping decisively out of my head. It wasn't till the top pulled out that I realized I'd been watching someone I'd heard about but had assumed was an urban legend. The fister, see, was an amputee missing most all of his lower arm, only too happy to slide his greased-up stump into a stud in a sling. Ah, those were innocent times.

I've never been fisted, and I doubt I ever will. It's not that it doesn't interest me. When I watch a bottom in ecstasy, I get envious. "It's unlike anything else. A feeling of total fullness, absolutely great," one fistee told me. But I guess I'll take his word for that, at least in this lifetime. A couple of hands have made it in me up to the knuckles, but I'm not planning on anything more extreme, not even from a munchkin in leathers.

And I'm really only a very occasional fisting top. Inserting hand into butt is one of those activities that, for me, has limited heat in and of itself. Handballing only gets me off if I'm really attracted to the guy in question. For whatever reason, there are fewer men I'd want to fist than I'd want to spank or tie up or fuck or suck off. I prefer my fistees to be somehow innocent-looking or ordinary—like the *Breakfast at Tiffany's* banker. Nothing too obviously sex-piggy. I guess it has something to do with violation.

Having my forearm jammed up a hot, wet space hasn't always been my idea of sexual fun; it took a while for me to figure out how I could really enjoy sticking my arm inside a guy. After all, the bottomboy was the one wallowing in sensation, and I was doing all the work. There's nothing particularly erotic, at least to me, in feeling my latex-shrouded hand mucking about in mucus membrane. But somewhere along the line I realized that if I got myself into a semi-sadistic mind space, the queasy combination of trust and trespassing involved in handballing could get my dick hard. If I look at it as a magical operation, one where I'm entrusted with a guy's fragile insides, then the power of it all shoots straight to my crotch.

I'm not the only one to see the magic in handballing. Years ago a wonderfully foo-foo book called *The Divine Androgyne* portrayed fist fucking as a high form of yoga, and I suppose that's accurate; never has butthole seemed more holy. There's definitely something mind-expanding the first time you see an arm slide inside. In fact, the whole notion of Sex Magic, of perversion as nirvana, is an interesting one, if a shade defensive. What was once regarded as sin—sin on a grand, deadly level—

has now been transmogrified through the efforts of a brave bunch of butt-fuck pioneers into a Search for Truth. Still, I've known plenty of guys who've done their time in a sling, and they, cross-sectionally, don't seem any more enlightened than your average, everyday sexpig. But their assholes sure are well-trained.

I confess: I'm of a generation that truly believed in the redemptive power of altered consciousness, so I'll probably go to my grave believing that there are whole marvelous realms of awareness that deserve to be explored. For a while it appeared that drugs would do the trick. Then, somewhere around the time of the Manson Family, we began to suspect that LSD might not be the one-size-liberates-all panacea that Tim Leary had made it out to be. In the meantime, the sexual kind-of-revolution and the rise of gay liberation brought sexual experimentalism to the forefront, at least within certain cock-hungry circles. And so it came to pass: The rise of S/M and the birth of the Modern Primitive movement popularized kink-as-spiritual-quest. What was "sick" had now become "sacred," in an oft-amusing blend of the piggy and the pious. When the Radical Faeries weren't prancing around in dresses, they were engaging in flesh-mortifying rituals formerly limited to a picturesque band of South Indian *sadhus*.

What with all the chitchat about endorphins, tribalism, and the dark search for transcendence, many twisted folks, not quite resigned to the dysfunctional truths of their kinkiness, have embarked on a quest to rationalize the irrational. Fisting can't just be crazy fun; it has to be *for* something. It's as if we pervs haven't quite shaken free of the Great Heteronormative Imperative: "Thou Shalt (Re)produce."

Raunch needs a reason, perversion an excuse. An urge, say, to drink pee can't simply be indulged: It's gotta be, in some way or another, *all right*. So there's a surfeit of pro-S/M propaganda about how kinkiness is just another harmless choice and how "safe, sane, and consensual" things are. But if we were to look the beast squarely in the eye, all but the most deluded of us would have to confess that while kink play should indeed be safe and consensual (or at least mostly so), it's hard to think of a grown man, naked except for a dog collar, crouching in a cage and eating Puppy Chow from a bowl as totally "sane." OK, it's not full-fledged bullgoose loony psychosis, but it is, to the dispassionate viewer, at least a little weird.

And there's nothing wrong with weird.

In fact, one might argue (and I'll give it a try) that the "stupid pervert," the one mindlessly jacking off into a pile of underwear, is actually more in tune with himself—possible guilt feelings and all—than the S/M liberals who twist themselves into knots explaining how it's all just good clean fun, as long as no one gets hurt more than he's agreed to. That's the problem with post-modern politics; it's damn near impossible to have good *dirty* fun anymore.

And then there are the sex police, whether well-meaning old-line lesbians or hard-shell Baptists, who use S/M as a bogeyman in chaps. *It's antihumanist, it's antiwoman, it's the Antichrist!* When confronted by the anti-kink forces, all one should have to do is stand up on one's hind legs and shout, "Listen, you meddling assholes, it's my fucking body and I'll do what I like with it, and if you disapprove…well, nobody's asking *you* to be tied to the St. Andrew's cross, now, are they?" And that should, in a just society, be that. Still, framing the debate in nice, nonthreatening terms may be vaccine against repression, or so we all hope, so I surely do appreciate the motivations of the S/M evangelists, those happy-face perverts who, instead of peddling *The Watchtower*, carry ball stretchers door-to-door.

And repression may be closer than we think. The censorious, the piously liberal, and the zealously religious are all intent on saving us from ourselves, by force if necessary. In the notorious "Spanner case," a bunch of British leathermen who'd engaged in a bit of thoroughly consensual slap-and-tickle were busted for assault; in the case of the masochists, they were convicted of taking part in *their own assaults*. As my late friend Vincent used to say, "Donnez-moi un fucking break!"

OK, so being fisted isn't good for you. Done wrong, or sloppily, without gloves or under the influence of whatever, it can be more than a little perilous. I know once-devoted bottoms who, after many a year spent in the sling, have decided to slack off and give their butts a well-deserved rest. Nevertheless, hands keep going up holes. There are even limber folks who can fist-fuck themselves and still stand up afterwards. It can be done. I've seen it. I've even seen two hands in one ass, and those hands were mine. But let's face facts: Taking a hand or two up the butt, no matter how enjoyable or often or easily done, is still perhaps a bit extreme.

Extreme. There's the operative word, one that both attracts and repels. For some reason, no doubt buried deep within the more primordial parts in the lobes of our brains, the human animal craves physical excitement, the challenge of stretching our bodies to their limits. Running a marathon, bungee-jumping, having kinky sex. And fisting is the Mount Everest of perversion. Why stick a hand into a greased-up asshole? Because it's there.

There are those who appreciate kink as a pleasant pastime, like raising tropical fish. They revel in the details of fetish, well-equipped toy bags, and the finely tuned modalities of lust. They're the hobbyists of whoring.

And then there's the hard-core bunch—the shameless sensation junkies. They're the Dionysian army, the folks who'd stake their sanity on sex. *Only one fist up your ass?* they taunt. *Why not take two? Or a foot?* Of course, a guy can be both dabbler and demon—sometimes one, sometimes the other, sometimes both at the same time. It just makes the game more complex, more fun. *How close to the edge can you get?*

The whole notion of losing control over lust gets some folks up in arms. The United States is still, underneath the constant merchandising of boobs and booty, a nation with Puritan roots. Throwing off self-respect and self-consciousness, and wallowing in the pleasures of the moment, seems somehow un-American. The Modern Primitives, with their hipper-than-thou Maori tattoos and genital piercings, are quite right about at least one thing: Being overcivilized can be a drag. And, in fact, kinky sex, both fisting and otherwise, can provide a way out. It's pleasure that isn't tied to the approved modes of sexual bonding, that sidesteps the tyranny of the penis and aims toward something else, and perhaps something new.

The first time I saw Fakir Musafar, who's generally recognized as one of the great pioneers of modern body modification, was at a hip-oisie preview of a documentary called *Dances Sacred and Profane* way back in the mid 1980s. Everyone in the audience was dressed in black. The film showed him performing the Native American Sun Dance. Fakir—a mild enough–looking fellow despite nipple piercings you could drive a truck through and a taste for astonishing corsets—got suspended by flesh hooks stuck through piercings in his chest. It was all fascinating, in a freak-show way. I was too hip to be repelled, too cool to be shocked. Little did I suspect that Fakir Musafar would someday become a friend, even supervising my few meager piercings, and that I'd get to know the filmmaker Charles Gatewood too. But most of all, I had no inkling of the coming boom in piercings, tattoos, and brandings. Who back then could anticipate that the kavadi, a pointed-sticks-in-flesh mortification ritual perfected somewhere near Calcutta, would become a craze in certain specialized circles, a Hula Hoop for the deeply twisted? That street fairs would feature entertainment by Ye Olde English Morris dancers with jingling bells hung from hooks through their skin? Who knew you'd be able to get your dick pierced on Main Street?

Just when the world was going virtual, when we all were shuffling off into cyberspace, there arose an urge for physical connectedness—for new, sometimes startling ways to get in touch with one's own body. Like the rise of fundamentalism, and the flowering of hippie culture before it, the Modern Primitive movement employed traditional means to sidestep the alienations of the modern world. There's something about challenging the body, whether atop a mountain, on a roller coaster, or in a sling, that gets us in touch with what we are. Fisting can do that. And, as with riding roller coasters, there arises in some kinksters the urge to go higher, faster, steeper.

It can be a problem. My youngish buddy Kent is concerned that he's getting habituated to S/M; that, addictlike, he's requiring edgier and edgier play to get him off. "Where will it end?" he asks, somewhat plaintively. And it's a valid question. Everyone, unless they're utterly psychotic, has limits. "And what if plain old nice sex is never enough for me again?" I would have liked to reassure him, tell him everything was going to be fine, but I was rather preoccupied with the imagined vision of him standing naked in big black boots, and me on my belly, licking the studded soles.

And so goes the search for more and more kicks, the bigger high. While most guys are happy to settle for vanilla, others for an occasional bit of perversion, some are so into their specific kink that nothing else can fully get them off. It's the textbook definition of a full-fledged fetish—a kink that's necessary for someone's sexual fulfillment. And, without sounding like someone's uptight aunt here, I'm not so sure that that level of obses-sion is all that healthy. Which is not to say that consensual, hard-core, balls-out, gotta-have-it fetishism should be a cause for tut-tutting disapproval, just that it seems kind of limiting, like being a crackhead or a Mormon.

"The world is so full of a number of things," says *A Child's Garden of Verses*, "I'm sure we should all be as happy as kings." Or queens. But if you absolutely *need* to suck on a tasseled loafer in order to come, that sort of narrows down the possibilities, no? Extreme fetishism has the romantic appeal of drug addiction or religious fanaticism: It orders the world around one imperative, one focus, one need. It simplifies things. And it gives you a ready-made community of sorts to relate to. But too much time spent on any one of the byways of desire, whether fist fucking or bondage or cock-and-ball torture, can have its pitfalls. Extremism in the pursuit of pleasure is no vice, but not everyone can stand the pace. I'm not being judgmental, but let's face facts—behind the delightfully obsessed kinkster can lurk a dam-aged soul. Holly Golightly might have been a charmingly off-kilter eccentric, but her creator, Truman Capote, was pretty much a fucked-up mess.

And when it comes to mess, there's not much potentially messier than a nice, long fisting session. Fisting is rarely an off-the-cuff diversion and is most emphatically not for the overly fastidious. There's the whole ritual of prior colonic clean-out, even a high-fat, low-fiber diet the day before to ensure slower movement down below; it's the perv's equivalent of carbo-loading. And even then, things get gooey. If any one kind of sex play most reminds us that we're meatbags with minds, it's fist fucking. Wallowing around in someone's colon may not sound transcendent or romantic or even very nice.

It is, indeed, a very strange yoga.

And yet, when my hand is deep within someone, when his eyes roll back and he moans in ecstasy and cum starts leaking out of his cock, when he maybe pisses himself, when I play with the fragility of the human animal, trespassing so deep I can feel the guy's heartbeat...

Well, it's fucking amazing—irrationally, transcendentally, disgustingly, gorgeously amazing. And there's nothing wrong with that.

CHAPTER 5
Sticks and Stones: Verbal Abuse

You fucking cocksucking faggot whore.

It's music to some guys' ears. Like Syd, a willowy, long-haired Asian guy in his late 30s. He and I have negotiated our scene earlier in the day, so when I show up and barge my way into his bedroom, wearing nothing but my chaps and boots, there he is face-down on the bed, naked except for women's high heels and fishnet stockings, more than ready to be treated like the pussyboy slut we've both agreed he is.

"You fucking piece of shit," I growl.

"Oh, yeah," he murmurs, humping the mattress. "Tell me what you're going to do to me."

As you might have gleaned by now, I take direction well. I begin to spin out a colorful tale of how I was going to rape his worthless slutpussy ass till he screamed.

"Say it louder."

I start to bellow abuse as the naked man in fishnets squirms.

"I'll do anything for you."

Yeah yeah, I think. As flattering as the notion might be, I've heard that line much too often to believe it.

"You'd better, you fucking cunt!" There! I've crossed the line and used the *c* word. Syd rolls onto his back, visibly aroused.

"Kill me," Syd coos.

But we've just met, I long to say. But I don't. I'm so well-behaved.

Instead, I launch into something I'd carefully talked over with him—a little eroticized racism. I tell him that he's my yellow bastard son, born of the cheap gook whore I fucked during my tour of duty in the Vietnam War.

He doesn't miss a beat. "Oh yeahhh…"

And so it goes, me fucking his face, him snorting head-splitting quantities of poppers, till he comes (three times, he'll tell me, although I really hadn't noticed) and I've shot off onto his smooth belly. All the while I've spewed a stream of insult and abuse. And he really liked that. Really.

After we've wiped up, we chat pleasantly for a while and then I head for home. Am I feeling ambivalent? Hmmm. Well, maybe.

Now, it's all well and good to write off scenes like this one as a harmless bit of fun, and indeed on one level they are. Only the stodgiest spoilsport would be unwilling to growl "You cocksucking pussyboy faggot" to a guy who is manifestly, well, a cocksucking pussyboy faggot. But the question of why both partners in these little tangos of verbal abuse should find their dicks hard and dripping is an interesting one.

I wasn't always into verbal abuse. I was first drawn into it, as is often the case with disreputable fun, by a fun-loving bottom looking for a top. Many years ago, I went home from a bar with a nice enough bloke who'd asked me to say nasty things while I fucked his face and pissed in his mouth. Easy enough for someone with my verbal facility, I figured. But in the event, it turned out that verbal assault wasn't the cinch I'd anticipated. The problem (besides trying to keep up a nice line of chat while being distracted by expert fellatio) was that there's a finite number of sufficiently nasty things to say. I ran through the basics fairly quickly, and then, to my chagrin, I started repeating myself. Take it from me: There's nothing worse than a budding V.A. top getting tongue-tied.

I did squeak through the scene without the bottom laughing. In fact, he rather enjoyed himself. And from then on, I started dabbling in the gentle art of eroticized insult. That's not to say I didn't have qualms; it was a leap for someone who came of age with the gay liberation movement to sling homophobic insults for fun…and to find it hot as fuck. I was hip to the notion of transgression, of course, and knew that in a mutually consensual scene, just about anything was fine and dandy. At least in theory. Regardless, I felt sullied. The question, as is the case with so much of queer kink, runs: Is this stuff a healthy release, a cathartic refashioning of oppression, turning homophobia into heat? Or is it a weird holdover from the bad old days, replaying anti-gay scripts that would just as well be left alone and forgotten?

Qualms, yes. But I didn't let them stop me. Eventually I started steering my verbal abuse from the cliché-filled highway of homophobia onto even more dubious side roads. From the commonality of queerness, I moved into the truly personal. Large guys became "fat," then "fat fags." The less endowed had "pathetic, tiny dicks." I played the race card. The religion card. And bingo, the bottoms enjoyed it.

So what the hell, I began to wonder, makes humiliation and degradation so damn hot for some of us? Whether taking abuse or dishing it out, are we thoroughly self-hating homos in need of psychiatric help? Or are we in some sense performing alchemy, turning crap into gold?

OK, so one of the goals of sex is ego loss, letting go—letting go of self-consciousness, our sense of self, maybe surrendering self-respect. Civilization has built up so much moralism around the simple squirting of seed that it's an unimaginative guy indeed who doesn't want to tear it all down. To have it battered down. To become, if only for a moment, pure flesh and desire, untouched by society and sense. It's why people get drunk, try drugs, do meditation or mutual masturbation—to get beyond the borders of the self, a self few of us are thoroughly comfortable with. And when you grow up queer in a queer-hating world, self-respect is a two-edged commodity. To access our deepest desires, we have to accept the fact that we're what the world despises: homos. So being told, convincingly, that we're twisted pigs has an oddly liberating effect. Because that's what we fucking are.

Words have always had a magically incantory effect, and that goes in spades for sex words. Maybe in the beginning the Word was with God, but it rapidly slipped below the belt. As part of a humiliation scene, a barrage of words filled with contempt and control can sure as shit be a shortcut to ecstasy, unlocking all sorts of lovely, squirmy, scary places. The more fastidious among us may find a date that includes placing one's head in the metaphorical toilet to be a bit declassé. And who am I, really, to argue? I can only protest that some of us do indeed get off on sex-as-Walpurgisnacht.

In these scenes of abasement and degradation, the script usually requires the top to "force" the bottom into submission. But, assuming the scene is consensual and not some prosecutable act, it's clear that whatever happens to Mr. Bottom Pussyboy is something he in fact hungers for. Far from shoving the kinky bottom into the gutter, the good (or at least smart) top realizes that he's providing the pretext for the submissive, a.k.a. "the sub," to crawl there on his own. Most of the time, the putative Nasty Master is not so much a slave driver as a tour guide, though it might take some of the fun away to acknowledge that. At a certain delightful point, though, the text and the metatext merge. Which is to say, in a less pretentious way, that a bottom may get off by "playing" a sick, twisted faggot slut, but who except a sick, twisted F.S. would get off on that kind of thing, anyway? Q.E.D. Did I truly want to fuck Syd up? Did I think of him as a cunt? Well, let's put it this way: Who but a cunt would leave the front door open so a complete stranger could clomp upstairs and abuse his fishnet-clad body, right? Just my presence there pretty much proved that everything I said about him was true. And so on, right down the hall of mirrors.

When I top, I can step back and convince myself I'm doing all that twisted stuff for the bottomboy's benefit. But then comes that little click that lets out my inner sadist, testing the limits rambunctiously as a pit bull on a chain. With a hard-on. Do I feel guilty?

Yes. And no.

As usual, the power positions in this filthy little song and dance are more complicated than the (somewhat appalled) casual observer might think. One reason I like to top in abuse and humiliation scenes is because I myself am far from a total top. I know the pleasure of huddling at a man's boots, licking the black leather clean. I know how lovely it can be to be treated as a worthless piece of meat, beneath the notice of a masterful, manly dom. I am, at times, a worthless cocksucking faggot myself, and if I can take another person to that sacred state, then the pleasure, both direct and vicarious, is mine. For when I give reign to my baser instincts, if only to drag a willing boy through the sewers of love, then where am I but in the sewers too?

It's the conundrum of being a conscientious sadist.

I always figured these qualms were pretty rare. But the other day, I was on the phone with a friend of mine, a handsome bisexual sadist in his mid 20s, the very model of the modern goth-boy top. It turned out that his favorite thing was, enchantingly enough, Red Army interrogation scenes, with him done up in a Soviet Army greatcoat and a chestful of medals. Just slipping on the drag made him hard.

Colin runs with a fairly interesting crowd: kids who set up orgies, take videos of the fuckfests, and later project the results at rave-ish dance parties. Sweet kids. Creative kids. The kind of twisted kids any parent would be proud to call his own. But Colin, though not yet 30, is kind of concerned about his sexual future. He worries that his Red Army kink is turning into a full-fledged fetish, that nothing short of the siege of Stalingrad will get his dick hard.

I can empathize. Fetishism, it seems to me, substitutes the part for the whole. What should be a broadening of sexual horizons can become a tightening shackle, a noose of nookie. I'd always figured that the more elaborate sorts of role-playing scenes were a ritualized cushion against the full impact of the basic joys of cruelty. The dog-and-pony show made things easier, safer. But hearing Goth Lad talk about it, I thought it was obvious that he shared, in some sense, my touchiness over just what he'd gotten himself into. Clearly, it wasn't enough of a crisis to merit his giving his Stalinist drag to the thrift store. There were too many bottoms out there hoping to be tossed into the gulag, and he was just the man to oblige. Nevertheless, he felt, as he put it, "Guilt. Well, not guilt exactly, but—"

"Ambivalence?" I offered.

"Yeah. I sometimes wonder just what I'm doing."

"I know what you mean," I said.

"See, I had this succession of girlfriends in college and…well, a lot of them were pretty fucked-up. One of them really liked abuse, had been abused as a child. She'd tried suicide. More than once."

I drew in my breath. I'd been lazily jacking off, thinking about this handsome guy, a young man I'd never played with and perhaps never would. Thinking about him dressed as a Commie commandant. Naked under a heavy Soviet greatcoat. Well, not totally naked. He'd be wearing boots, and I'd be groveling at his feet, hoping for a glimpse of his rampant rod. Maybe even hoping to get brutally fucked. Not that I was worthy. Not that I was the least bit worthy. He was young and handsome and ruthless. I just pretended to be cruel. He was the real thing. He was vital and strong, and the most I could hope for was to be his worthless supplicant. Oh yeah. Oh yeah. It was close enough to Workers' Paradise for me.

But then Colin mentioned the suicide attempts. My hand reflexively left my cock, though I remained hard, excited now to be taken into his confidence. By the thought of consequences.

It's easier to be a sick motherfucker when you ignore the notion of consequences. Even the heaviest S/M scene is self-contained, or so the story goes. People—sometimes people with low self-esteem, extreme neuroses, real problems—get spit on, cursed on, and beaten, and then everyone zips up and goes home. No harm done. Sticks and stones can break my bones, but words can never harm me.

Of course, I'd like to believe that everyone I've ever abused went away the better for the experience. After a scene I'll often ask "How're you doing?" That's what experienced players often do, though it might be more consistent with bottoms' fantasies if I just kicked them out the door and threw their clothes after them. Hell, maybe I'm just too nice for my own good.

After I played with one bottom, I worried about just that. He usually went for nominally straight guys who'd insult him, "force" him to wear panties, fuck his face, and tell him to get lost. Or so he said. But hell, I *liked* him, and I suppose that showed. So maybe having sex with some kindly old sadistic fag like me was unsatisfying, less humiliating than giving it up for some rotten straight buck would be. Or perhaps—and here's what gave me pause—it was in fact *more* humiliating. Oh dear.

Looking too deeply into the eroticization of degradation is simply too old-fashioned and pre-postmodern to bother with. It's all a game, of course, just a bit of harmless fun. Or so we'd like to think. But—and here's the terrifying, cool part—maybe not.

It's a puzzle, that borderline between healthy, consensual fun and dark neurosis. Are we cauterizing wounds or picking at the scabs till they bleed again? I'm glad my primary relationship isn't S/M–based; it might get too confusing to navigate the shoals of truth and desire.

I'm Instant Messaging a 20-year-old who calls himself "ricky"—a very beautiful, very skinny boy with a smallish dick. He craves abuse. He longs to lick the sweat from disdainful jocks.

"i was bullied in high school, pushed around. The school i went to was a small school, where sports dominated everything. i tried out, but i was too wimpy to make any of the teams. i was laughed at and called names."

"Well, at least," I type back, twisting the knife a bit, "they were paying attention to you."

"Yeah, at first i thought they liked me, but later figured out they didn't."

"Did being bullied make you hard?" I am genuinely, if sadistically, curious.

"Oh, yes, i got hard. It was impossible to control it."

"And now?"

"i just enjoy being humiliated and degraded. It helps me get off."

Obligingly I type away, calling him a sick sissy cunt, spinning out tales of hard-core humiliation and torture, threatening things I'd really at least consider doing to a boy so cute and needy. Needy. That's the rub. As we chat about my tying him to a post and leaving him to starve, the skinny boy getting even skinnier, weaker, pissing himself, fainting, Colin's qualms come to mind. Here is a young man with—clearly—Issues. He's been victimized by machismo and homophobia, things I despise. And here I am replaying those sad scripts, eroticizing the pain. Am I a healer? Or a monster? And if I am indeed a monster, does my achingly hard hard-on make matters better or worse?

Many of us fags harbor fantasies of revenge, ways to get back at those fucking high school bullies, the ones who grow up into right-wing politicians and homophobic preachers, the assholes who hurt us for no fucking good reason. Kink, for better or worse, allows us take that aggression out on one another, on ourselves, instead. If this were a just world, someone would tie up and torture those bastards who made ricky's youth a misery. Unlike the pleasing symmetries of S/M porn stories, in real life ricky's tormentors most likely wouldn't enjoy being worked over by a leatherman with a whip. Not a bit.

And if I weren't such a sick fuck, I would, like some leather Virgin Mary in a prurient pietà, be metaphorically stroking ricky's lovely face, a healing touch with no taint of violence.

I'd be hard-pressed to defend how *wrong* I thought he was to eroticize his own misery. And yet what alternatives are there? Years of therapy at 100 bucks an hour? Actually wreaking revenge on his erstwhile tormentors in some lurid movie-of-the-week scenario? His becoming a sadist himself someday and taking it all out on willing young men?

But then, if the bullies hadn't picked on ricky, I never would have been chatting with him. If I didn't have at least a smidgen of bully in me, I never would have popped a woody when I read his online profile. Our dicks wouldn't have been hard as we planned on my making him into a human toilet. We were, he and I, complicit in our own oppression. Especially *his* oppression.

And that guilt—just between you and me—only made things hotter.

Hot. Very, very hot. Those of you not into it probably think of cyber contacts as hopelessly abstract and second-rate. But if the brain is, as the saying goes, the largest sexual organ, then ricky had given me a cerebral woody. Unmoored from our physical bodies, the contact we made was somehow more intense than face-to-face tricking might have been. Which is not to say that I didn't imagine, very concretely, working ricky over. Skinny ricky, his hands tied above his head, stretched-out body half-suspended from a beam. Little dick rock-hard. Skin-and-bones pussyboy ricky, being slapped around, degraded, pissed on for my amusement. Sure, something had gone wrong in his life, but why the fuck should I not be the one to take advantage of that?

For me at that moment, the connections between him and me, between ricky and the burden of his past, between me and my complex desires, all of that was shining and true. And as dangerous as shouting "fag" in a crowded bathhouse.

I've always believed that politics stops at the bedroom door. (Or at least I *thought* I believed that.) Play between consenting adults, whether sexist, racist, blasphemous, or just plain disgustingly nasty, should be nobody else's business. You want to play the lecherous uncle and the innocent young boy? Or the murderous rapist and the sleeping victim? For God's sake, do it. Just don't confuse fantasy and real life.

It might seem that consensual verbal abuse scenes pose far less danger than scenes in which canes, chains, or red-hot branding irons are involved. But names can indeed harm us; just ask anyone who's grown up being called "faggot." That is, I suppose, the reason so many folks who are into kink rely on ritual, heavy role-playing, uniforms of one sort or another. If you're playing with antisocial shit from your own damn past, a certain amount of buffering's not a bad idea. Like with ricky: Would I really do all the terrible things I'd contemptuously threatened, to his unmitigated delight? Well...maybe some of them. Maybe most of them. Maybe. I did tell him the truth when I said I wanted to punish him for his beauty, make him cry. But that wasn't all I wanted to punish him for. I wanted to punish him for making me want to punish him. I wanted to beat the pain out of both of us. And I wanted, oh sweet Buddha, to do something unforgivable.

There's such a big thrill in guilt and damnation. Whole religions, notably Roman You-know-what, are built on the thrill of dancing on the razor's edge of almost unforgivable sin. It's really no wonder, I guess, that so many priests turned out to be doing the dirty with little boys; short of murder, what else could they do that would lead them so directly to the darkness that lurks in all our damnable souls?

Poor ricky. If any perversion can be called poignant, it's his. He wanted love, he got abuse. And now, with my pledges to tie him up, spit on him, flog him, and then kiss him hard, I'm trying to make things all better. A Band-Aid on a beheading.

"I want to possess you totally...and give you everything you need," I type out, anxious not to be a total beast. I can see how battered wives could stay with their hubbies. In some awful way, even malevolent attention is better than none.

"i'd know you loved me as you used my body. Sir, own me mentally, physically, totally for your pleasure."

"You're a sick fuck, ricky."

"Very true, Sir. It's just what i enjoy. i learned to enjoy the bullying, and sometimes i think that i'm a fucked-up kid, but I don't know how to fix myself. i'm stuck this way, but i enjoy who i am."

Since our online meeting, I've thought of ricky often. Who knows; if he weren't in the Midwest and me in California, perhaps we'd meet, reality bumping up against our most extreme fantasies. For all I know, he's out there in Ohio, a well-adjusted, happy, self-possessed young man who likes to dabble in verbal abuse and walk away with a happy smile, while I, for my part, fret and feel guilty. I hope so. I really do.

CHAPTER 6

Acting With Restraint: Bondage

Handsome Ted was a bondage top with fabulous rope technique. I was his fan. I loved watching him in action at play parties. He was quick, he was skilled, and his tied-up bottoms always looked fabulous. I wanted someday to be as expert as Ted. I wanted him to teach me his technique. Well, actually, I wanted him to tie me up. And so one day—my birthday, as it happened—I popped the question. And Ted said yes, he'd put me in bondage. Oh joy, oh rapture, I was going to be tied up by a sexy expert! And at a dungeon party, no less!

I stood naked against the cold metal bars of a cage as Ted wound rope after rope around me: My outstretched arms got bound to the bars, then torso, legs, and ankles, rope snaking between my legs, around my thighs. It was not, for me, directly erotic. I'm not a true bondage bottom; the feeling of being restrained isn't, in itself, enough to make my penis hard. But it was, nevertheless, a wonderful feeling, being attended to so assiduously. That bottomy feeling of being the center of the universe was what gave me a woody.

At last, his handicraft complete, my very own bondage master stepped back, having done a job I could only aspire to. I stood, exposed to all, firmly tied up, the birthday boy in bondage. It was bliss. I struggled, ever so slightly, just to feel the ropes push back. And then… And then I felt the ropes around my crotch and thighs slowly but inexorably loosen, give way, start creeping slackly down my thighs. Surprise!

Ted didn't miss a beat; unfazed, he rejiggered the ropes till they were once again taut. He knew he was good. He knew he was in control. He didn't have to bluster and strut to prove it. No muss, no fuss, no ego. Sometimes a birthday present is unexpected but nonetheless precious for all that. And since then I've aspired to Tedhood.

Back when I was a just slightly experienced kinkster, I went to bondage classes, which was even more California than it sounds. There I was, like some slightly demented Boy Scout earning his Perversion Merit Badge: observing, taking notes, then practicing knots and rope handcuffs on my partner during the workshop session. As hokey as it may have seemed, I learned a lot from Restraints 101. There's not, it turns out, just one type of bondage. Of course not. As with every area of erotic specialization, there are numerous subtle variations. There's American-style bondage, the most familiar kind, in which fairly short lengths of rope are used to bind together wrists or ankles, or to tie a victim to a snazzy bondage board or a plain old chair. On the other hand, Japanese-style bondage uses longer ropes, often 25 feet or more, to enmesh the body in a continuous webwork. Those of us who are bondage aficionados simply love the look of flesh in ropes, and each variation, be it Bettie Page or Bangkok whorehouse, offers its own aesthetic pleasures.

Bondage, especially the fancier sort, is about control, sure, but it's also about decor. Like getting dressed up in fetish clothing, bondage is costuming for the sex show. A lot of high-end bondage porn features photo spreads remarkable for their melodramatic perfection, though, sad to say, some of it isn't functional at all. Attempting to duplicate the intricate ropework seen in *Bound and Gagged* magazine more often than not results in a puzzled-looking bottom and a pile of clothesline on the floor.

Contrivance? Sure, but what is bondage gear but a collection of contrivances?

Depending on the skill and ambition of the top, rope bondage can be largely symbolic, or damn near inescapable, or even stressful, stretching the bottom's body into clearly uncomfortable positions. My first teacher was into elaborate Japanese-style bondage, macramé for the masochist. So we learned an arms-behind-the-back number supposedly used in samurai days to restrain the shogun's prisoners. And we were taught to make a lovely rope body harness, knotted webwork stretching from shoulders to crotch that enclosed the torso in a latticework of rope. Yum. I could barely wait to try it out on someone besides the bored and boring straight guy who served as my practice bottom.

When I got home with my metaphorical merit badge and hastily scrawled notes, I set out to practice what I'd been taught. I got my boyfriend to stand still long enough to try tying him up, but damn, it was tough to reconstruct all those elaborate twists and turns. In the weeks that followed I tried my skills on a number of willing victims. Some of it worked, some of it didn't. Bondage, especially rope bondage, turns out to be a matter of problem-solving. And sometimes I ended up just plain flummoxed.

So of course, like any eternal student, I went back to school. I took another bondage class, this one taught by a burly guy whose approach was, he professed, "quick and dirty." Unlike the previous teacher and his ultra-aesthetic approach, this one said, "I'm a lazy top. I want to get them tied up quickly and securely so I can use 'em." Which seemed sensible to me. His rope harness was not only a lot easier to put on, it could be undone without 10 minutes of detangling. Suddenly, there was no *right* way to tie someone up. I liked that.

And I liked tying up a variety of usually naked, usually quite hard men.

Playing top in a bondage scene, I came to realize, can be just like putting on a show. If it's a one-on-one, then the drama's for an audience of a single guy, the ever eager-to-be-entertained bottom. But there are things about restraint scenes—the decorative nature of the art, the thrill of being helpless in front of others, a top's pride in his arts-and-crafts handiwork—that fairly beg for public display. I've seen plenty of gorgeous bondage at S/M parties, some of it accomplished enough to make me feel a tad inadequate, though—not to boast—I've received my share of praise as well. OK, so tying a guy up isn't rocket science. Still, there's something about the flexibility of flesh that makes secure and tidy bondage a bit of a challenge. You can spend a lot of time and effort getting things just right, working for symmetry, tucking in every end, standing back in self-congratulation, only to watch as those ropes go slack, slide around, droop. It can get frustrating, and more so if there's a cluster of horny men watching. (And at times like that, it's good to remember Ted.)

Things are easier when using a bondage table or other secure tie-down point rather than just tying up a freestanding boy, but there's always an element of technique when it comes to rope. Needless to say, consumer capitalism has produced a near-endless line of gadgets to assist in the gentle art of restraint: metal shackles, bondage mitts, amazing straps and clasps, lots and lots of stuff. But I want to be loved for what I know, not for what I own. I don't even crave an SUV, not even one with a naked boy in the back. I guess I'm just not a good American.

When it comes to libidinal curry, restraint can be the bit of lime pickle that spices things up; rare is the bottom, no matter how vanilla, who doesn't love to have his wrists pinned to the bed. But for others, bondage is a big spicy dish in itself. Some guys are into bondage as the main course, others as a prelude to other things—spanking, fucking, cock milking, foot worship, you name it. I generally prefer to use the bondage within a larger scenario. Things can be basic: You tie him up and fuck him. Or more baroque, as when I tied one yuppie in boxer shorts to a chair, hands behind his back, legs spread wide, then grabbed a big old pair of scissors and, as prearranged, slowly sliced into his Brooks Brothers undies until his hard dot-com cock emerged from the shredded cotton. As he strained against the ropes, I drew the business end of the blade across his oh-so-tender, suddenly damp dickflesh. I looked into his blandly handsome face. *I didn't cut you*, I thought, *but I fucking could have.* When I looked down again, his creamy load had, irresistibly, oozed out of his endangered dick. It's shivery moments like that that make learning square knots worthwhile.

It's possible to play out very scary, brutal bondage scenes, of course. But there's a sweet paradox to bondage: What looks like danger can feel like safety. Even when the play's awash in edgy threat and vulnerability, the embrace of rope and restraints is, often as not, oddly comforting. While it's possible to just clamp some leather restraints on wrists and ankles and call it a day, rope bondage is usually a rather leisurely, caring pursuit. It's kink for patient perverts, the *tai chi* of sex. I've always found the experience of being a bondage bottom delightfully indulgent, kicking back as some diligent top makes sure my body is well attended to. It's what I imagine a trip to a luxury spa would be like, assuming that all around you men were being spanked and tortured.

Total bondage scenes, where the restraint is the ultimate end in itself, has a weird, unexpected purity—Zen with an erection. The limitations of the flesh fall away. OK, I'm veering perilously close to the "magical" model of S/M here, but there does seem to be something near-meditative about a lot of bondage scenes, kind of like the sensory deprivation tanks that were once all the New Age rage.

This is especially true of total immobilization scenes, the kind that can involve pricey full-body leather "sleep sacks" or cheap-but-effective mummification with Saran Wrap and duct tape. Years ago I took part in a group scene where a naked man was enclosed in one of those leather sacks, just a piece of meat in polished cowhide, and suspended on tippy-toes from a hook in the ceiling. Four of us unsnapped flaps over his nipples and dick, torturing his tits and cock and paddling his butt. It was fun, in a club-the-piñata way, but fairly well removed from what I find sexy. Its appeal would probably become apparent to me if I got laced up into a sleep sack myself, but I guess I'm too cowardly—or claustrophobic—to seek a top with the equipment. A well-to-do top, because those sleep sacks are expensive: Custom-made models cost thousands of bucks. Actually, *all* that bondage junk is pricey, from cast-iron shackles to delightful gizmos of leather and chain. It is a specialty market, after all, and the mass production of latex masks with piss tubes is unlikely to make anyone as rich as Henry Ford. Just walking into a leather store is sufficient to remind me how many geegaws I'll never be able to afford. It's enough to give a guy a case of equipment envy. But even a pair of the cheesiest handcuffs can do wonders for someone's state of mind. The ratchets click, the metal tightens down, the dick gets hard. *You have the right to remain silent…*

We all, at some point or another, want—no, *need*—to feel powerless in the grip of something just plain *more* than ourselves. Whether that something is love, religion, or shiny new manacles from the local leather store depends on the luck of the draw. Matter of fact, my brilliant editor at Alyson pointed out that bondage is religious in the most literal sense of the word: *Religare* means "to constrain" or "to bind together."

The reassuring security of helplessness harkens back, perhaps, to childhood; the well-loved rugrat is so powerless, so cared for, so safe. Ah, to return to that infantile Eden. (Actually, my bondage-top fantasies go way back too. I was a kid during the golden age of gladiator movies—Steve Reeves, not Russell Crowe. I vividly remember altering the newspaper ads for such cinema classics as *Hercules Unchained*, erasing bit of loincloth, adding more ropes, transforming the dubbed, protohunky actors in the sword-and-sandal epics into my very own sex toys. This primitive Photoshop gave me virtual possession of something I must have figured I'd never actually lay my hands on: sexy, semi-naked, tied-up men. Well, I was wrong.)

Conversely, being a bondage top is sorta like being a parent. Or God. You look upon a (more or less) naked form, decide that it is good, then tie it the hell up. Your own private Adam, at the mercy of…well, you.

Bondage can be read (on a pretentiously symbolic level, natch) as the physicalization of deeper struggles. Being captured by lust, conquered by another man's attractiveness. Being enslaved, in fact, by your own desires. Cowhide and rope encase the body. Human flesh encases the heart. It's all, in its way, beautiful and poignant. Yes, poignant. These are, admittedly, pretty abstract thoughts when you've got someone hog-tied and helpless in your bed and you reach down to his semi-helpless body, slide your fingers between his ass cheeks, and feel the heat from within. But stick with me, OK? Don't force me to do something I'll "regret."

Some of the paradoxical freedom experienced by bondage bottoms comes from the granting of permission. Being tied up in a pain scene keeps you from squirming away from what you, in fact, want to happen. Being tied up in a cock-milking scene puts your orgasm, literally, in another man's hands. Though restraint may from the outside seem arduous, it is, in a sense, the submissive's Easy Way Out. Inner conflicts are externalized, ritualized, neatened up in a consensual bit of playacting. Got second thoughts? You don't have to deal with them; your Master will. Absolved of responsibility, you can just lie back, unable to budge, and enjoy yourself.

It's all part of the central conundrum of consensual S/M. The tied-up bottomboy would appear not to have any choice. He's "helpless," compelled to do precisely the things he most desires to do. When a sub says "I want you to force me to…" just what does that mean? What *can* it mean? It means "I want you to pretend to force me," of course, but more crucially, "I want to pretend I don't want you to do these things to me." By colluding with this basic bit of dishonesty, the nice old top takes things even further from the truth of the matter, letting the bottom off easy. The bottom, around whose twisted, dirty longings (let's face it) the whole scene revolves, is given back his innocence, phony as it may be.

The top, meanwhile, is in a whole other space, "controlling" but being controlled by the bottom's desires. BDSM scenes may indeed be collaborations, symbiotic moments of need and fulfillment, meetings between slavering pigboys and sneering Masters. And yet, despite the consensuality, the mutuality of it all, there is a real gap, perhaps unbridgeable, between the top's and bottom's positions. The top is the alchemist, but more than that, he's the detective, the explorer, the miner who brings forth what was hidden, forcing the issue. The bottom is the ground of desire but also that which must be excavated, violated. Sure, all the role-playing may indeed be a bogus dumb-show, a well-enacted scene of Let's Pretend. Yet on a deeper level, maybe what *seems* to be happening is in fact what really *is* happening. A subversive idea, perhaps, but one that keeps kink as dangerously absorbing as we'd all like it to be. It's what, I can't help feeling, makes the whole song and dance worthwhile. Whoa, dude, it's for real!

Those ropes and padlocks only make palpable a power relation that's already been mutually agreed on. It's less demeaning, less radical, less submissive for a bottom to struggle against real chains than to be bound only by his willingness to submit. And as we all kind of know already, the most restrictive bonds are the ones inside each of us. The best, strongest, kinkiest restraints are those in the mind.

It took just one very intense scene to convince me of how hot that fact could be. He was the sadistic top, I was his maso-bottom. He slapped me with a leather strap that hurt like hell, and hey, my limits aren't the highest. So things might have gone easier if he had tied me down. But he didn't believe in making things easy for me. I was naked, no ropes, no restraints, wearing nothing but a hard-on and a (most likely) anxious expression.

"Lie there," he said, "and don't move a fucking muscle." And the strap came down. I tried not to shy away. "Stay STILL, damn it!" and the strap came down again. I struggled not to struggle. And again. "That's it, boy. Still. Do your fucking best. Do it for me." The pain was tough to take, but the inner struggle was 10 times worse. I wanted to thrash around, protect myself. After a while I wanted to rear back and punch him. Instead, with his stern encouragement, I stayed as still as I could. For him. And for me.

He was such a damn good top, reading my reactions, knowing when I'd approached my (to me, too wimpy) limits, when to slack off, perhaps stroke my aching ass, and when to let me have it again. He was handsome, he was powerful, but what kept my dick hard was something else, something more important. Something dark and private and very, very real.

At last, knowing I'd taken as much as I could, he released me.

Not from mere rope, but from myself. As he took me in his arms and stroked my face, as he kissed my tears away and gave me back myself, I realized I'd been taught a lesson by a masterful Master.

Wherever you are, Sir, thank you.

CHAPTER 7

Ouch! Pain Play

We'd met at a sleazy bar. He was visiting from Boston, good-looking in a nerdy sort of way, and he was into biting. Big time.

I was in a "What the hell?" mood, so I'd invited him over.

He had me naked on the bed, his sharp little teeth making painful excursions to my underarms, inner thighs, neck. Biting down. Ow. It hurt. It really hurt. Unlike spanking, flogging, or cock-and-ball torture, it was not a sensation that I found even remotely pleasurable. And he just kept on nibbling. Bite, bite, bite, less like an Anne Rice story than like being trapped with a gaggle of starving rats.

Part of me wanted to tell him to stop, command him to stop, to knee him in his groin and then shove him out the door. I didn't though. Because, I wondered, *If this is so painfully unerotic, then why the hell is my dick so hard?*

Days later, long after I'd cum, he'd cum, he'd gone back to Boston, and the nasty yellowish bite-shaped bruises all over my poor body were starting to fade, I was still wondering the same thing.

Years later, I'm hanging out with a buddy in Dolores Park. It's a sunny day. Richard is excited because he's just spent the night with this guy he's been seeing, a muscular little hottie. And, Richard says, they've been getting into some really hot fighting scenes. He pulls off his jacket to show me the bruise on his biceps, then happily pulls up his shirt; his lean body is bruised where, he says cheerfully, his play buddy's fists have landed.

"God," he says, "it's so nasty, and it hurts, and I'm having so much fun." So much fun, in fact, that he was semi-laid-up for a day or two when one of their sessions got a bit out of hand. But he's proud of it all, in a weird way. It's proof he can take it. It's clear he has a big crush on the guy, who he describes as scrappily good-looking in a slightly disreputable, rough-trade way. The more he talks about the somewhat brutal object of his affection, the more I suspect I know him.

Finally, I ask, "You don't have to say anything if you don't want to, but is it Bret?"

"Yeah," Richard says with a sheepish-but-proud grin. "You know him?"

As it happens, I do. Bret and I have occasionally kneed each other's balls. Cock-and-ball torture has never been a favorite of mine; I find the vulnerability of a guy's nuts a little scary, and having my own worked over has always been more queasy-making and cringe-producing than erotic. That is, until I met Bret, a tough-looking longhair with a tight, muscular body. (And, as it happened, big, meaty, low-hanging balls.) At first I went through with the CBT just so I could get to play with Bret, whose streetwise attitude fascinated me. He, on the other hand, liked me for my sadistic streak. "There's something hot," he'd say, "about having my nuts hurt by a man who's older and not as strong as I am." Well, I sure wasn't about to argue with him about that.

Bret liked to strut his toughness; he'd participated in a lot of wrestling scenes, both sexual and not, and he really was a butch bit of work. But he also enjoyed it when I zeroed in on his most vulnerable spot and made him wince. Most younger guys, he told me, seemed to want to hold back. It was the older ones who were nasty enough to let his nuts have it.

Conversely, if I was going to let anyone make my testicles hurt, Bret was clearly high on the list. And so we'd meet at his place, drop our trousers, stand face-to-face just inches apart, and make each other's genitals ache. Keeping up with him was quite a challenge. He was a total switch who liked to give as good as he got, and he could take quite a lot and still keep grinning. I let him do things to me no one else ever had, like get me on all fours and attack my ball sac from behind. In the abstract, it seemed too risky and not much fun, but when it came time to grind our heels into each other's private parts, it always turned out to be amazingly exciting. Sure, there are plenty of tests of endurance, but not all of them produce hard-ons.

The thing to keep in mind about sadomasochism is that it really *is* about pain. Sometimes that gets lost amidst the palaver about negotiations, safewords, and the production of endorphins. But beyond the Modern Primitive schtick and the Mister Leather contests, an irreducible fact remains: For a significant number of people, hurt is sexy. Not all hurt, of course. As my friend Chris says, "Just because I'm a masochist, that doesn't mean I enjoy stubbing my toe." But for genuine sadomasochists, given the right context and a compatible partner, sex with pain is just plain better than sex without. And for a goodly proportion of those folks, pain can even serve as a stand-in for sex; many an S/M scene has nothing to do with the genitals at all.

Playing with pain is, to the civilian masses, either downright icky, or a bit titillating and more than a little sick. The normative world has tried to explain it away. Shrinks explore our upbringing. Academics natter on about the discourses of power in terms only they understand. Politicos blame it on the culture of violence, puritanical feminists on male hegemony or some damn thing. Meanwhile, S/M enthusiasts rhapsodize about endorphins and spiritual quests, burning sage in the four cardinal directions before beating the shit out of one another. And there's a grain of truth in all that stuff. But I've come to believe that none of these explanations really matters. Oh, they can help us understand what we feel, maybe. They can even provide a pretext for guilt or acceptance. But they can never fully explain sadism, masochism, and the sharp, chilly, ever-wavering border between the two. Because it's all a mystery. It really is. A dark, awful, fucked-up, shining mystery. And at a time in history where the last wild places on Earth are being McDonaldized, where everything transcendent is either rationalized away by science or made lapdog-manageable through the low-level use of religion, it's nice to know that the ultimate darkness is still within, that we can go there, and that no one can ever take that away—not Freud, not Jesus, not Andrea Dworkin. It's a contaminated pleasure, perhaps, but it's real and it's our own.

Maybe my sample is skewed, but sometimes I'm amazed at just how kinky the average queer guy seems to be. Ian, for example. I first met him on the street, all 6 foot 6 of him, when he was on his way to return a video.

He was tall. And cute. And tall. And when he spoke it was obvious he wasn't very butch, which was just fine with me. I already had to look up at him, way up, and if he'd been aggressive as well as that cute I might have lost my nerve. But he wasn't, I didn't, and several days later we ended up in my bed.

If Ian turned out to be somewhat more effeminate than I might have expected, he also turned out to be a hell of a lot more fun. He was, he'd said, pretty damn vanilla, but he was willing to give kink a whirl.

OK, so how about if I spanked him?

That would be fine, he said, turning his furry butt my way, ready to receive the impact of my hand. He wasn't the first spanking virgin I'd broken in, and I knew that when it turns out that a fella likes to be spanked, he usually likes to be spanked a *lot*. Ian did. A lot. And when he'd had enough, when his pretty ass was a gratifyingly bright pink and more-than-warm to the touch, I fucked it.

"Wowee!" he said, charmingly, after he'd cum. "That sure was amazing."

Well, perhaps not amazing, but nice. Very, very nice. Ian and I became fuck buddies, and I gently but firmly helped him discover just what a sick puppy he could be. Eventually, after intros to flogging, chest-slapping, and cock-and-ball torture, one day the libidinal tables got turned. With a puckish look, Ian slapped my scrotum. Now, any Total Top worth his salt would have bridled. And, my balls being pretty damn sensitive, it actually *hurt*.

I was delighted.

I was delighted at Ian's enterprise, his playfulness, his taking the time to figure me out and try something like that. To the tradition-bound eye, his flipping me might have seemed out of bounds, but it fit into the evolving relationship between us just fine.

Eventually, our buddyhood fizzled out. These things do. I didn't hear from him for half a year or more. But just the other week I was pleasantly surprised to get a phone call from him. Could he come over and play? Well, sure.

Turns out he's been through a lot of drama. He's found himself a new, pretty damn kinky boyfriend. Though he remains HIV-negative, he's been diagnosed with chronic hepatitis C, putting him in a new, more problematic relationship with his own body. And would I mind putting on my best boots and kicking his ass? Nope, I wouldn't mind, not I. So I do it, getting nastier with him than ever. I kick his butt, I step on his chest, I grind my heel into his hard-on. Ian leaves with a startling bruise on his dick and a big ol' smile on his face. We aim to please.

There are plenty of men out there who define themselves as Total Tops. It would hurt their pride, I guess, to admit they have even a teeny tiny bit of interest in being worked over. But I must lack moral fiber or something. I like to lie back and be beaten. After all, the rewards of topping in a pain scene are very different from the pleasures of bottoming.

Pain-scene bottoms are put in immediate touch with their bodies when they get spanked, caned, pierced, or what have you. Not only do they have immediate erotic responses to the hurt, they often acquire the skill to process pain, transforming what most of us would find uncomfortable, even unbearable, into intense but enjoyable sensation.

The top's enjoyment, though, is almost entirely vicarious. Spanking someone, dripping molten wax on their tits, or ranging clothespins along an engorged cock doesn't *feel* good, at least not physically, warm though it may the cockles of a sadist's dark heart. And the taking of joy from inflicting pain, no matter how consensual and negotiated and longed-for by the bottom, is a bit sick, no? You can pretty it up, dress it in gleaming leather, call it "sex magic" or "power exchange," but maybe those who tut-tut S/M have a point? Maybe the sadist stuff is somehow wrong? Immoral, even? Nah, couldn't be…

Things get even more trickily theatrical at S/M play parties, where guys are pretty literally onstage while they do all that nasty stuff. Not so long ago I was at a dungeon party, watching an extended flogging scene. The bottom, a handsome middle-aged guy in a jockstrap and boots, was bound facedown to an X-shaped St. Andrew's cross. The top, in jeans and a Harley T-shirt, looked tough as an ex-con—which, I had it on reliable information, he was.

"That's it, bitch," he growled, a big multitailed flogger in each hand. "Show me what you got." Again and again the floggers landed on the bottom's bright-red back, eliciting trembling, groans, yells. It was—there's no other word for it—brutal. I watched, mouth agape, feeling somewhat inadequate. Not only would I never, ever be able to stand even a fraction of the pain the bottom was soaking up, I wasn't even sure I'd want to dish out that level of abuse. Now, the rational part of me knows that life isn't a contest, like "He who dies with the most welts wins." Some homos, hard to believe as it may be, haven't ever even been spanked. Not even a gentle swat. Not once.

"Yeah, bitch. You had enough yet?" barked Mr. Ex-Con.

I didn't really find the scene sexually arousing. I found it…well…*interesting*. Even a bit, if I were to admit it to myself, off-putting. Still, the maso-guy was taking a hell of a lot, was obviously near his limits, and the scent of agony hung heavy in the air. I couldn't look away. And I noticed I wasn't alone: Half a dozen other guys were raptly watching the scene unfold. I found myself wondering about straight and dyke S/M; this was so obviously a very male-versus-male test of wills. Clearly, it was consensual play. And despite his criminal past (or maybe because of it), the top obviously knew what he was doing—his flogging technique was impeccable. But still, there was something about the scene that seemed, at least to me, at least that night, to be…evil. And just thinking in such moralistic, old-fashioned terms prompted a guilty little shiver of pleasure. I'm such a goddamn pervert.

"You had enough yet, bitch?"

At last, at last, the poor suffering bottom said "Yes."

"One more, then." The floggers went up. The floggers came

down—hard—on naked flesh. The top laid down his tools of torture, stepped to the man on the cross, and kissed and stroked his victim's battered flesh. The little crowd of spectators dispersed.

A bit later I overheard one of the other guys at the party, a fortyish man who specializes in being a "little boy" for his Daddies, talking about the scene. "Ooh," he cooed, "that man was just too mean for me." And who the hell was I to disagree?

There are certainly plenty of reasons to have sex, but one of the aims—OK, maybe *the* aim—of sex (good sex, anyway) is the loss of self-awareness, the transcendent moment when fleshly pleasure is all. S/M goes to great lengths to achieve this release, subjecting the body and soul to all sorts of extremes. Yet (and aye, here's the paradoxical rub) consensual S/M is in some sense always a performance, a played-out scene requiring heightened self-awareness to pull off. Eventually, of course, the Great Cosmic Fuckmelt can be reached, often is, but leathersex sure takes the long way 'round—setting up barriers of self-consciousness, then battering right through them.

That's certainly one reason why, for many men, S/M and drug use go hand in hand. Poppers—good poppers, anyway—provide ego loss on demand. Quick Roto-Rooter rushes give way to thoughts along the lines of "Well, here I am with my tongue up some guy's ass, and just how the hell did I *get* here, anyway?" And maybe a headache. More major drugs and/or booze provide other ways to slide past the limits of self-consciousness, but the road to dickly nirvana can be a twisty one, and playing when you're wrecked can be like trying to drive with a blindfold on. Wrecked, indeed.

Pain isn't the only sort of torture out there. Those of us who grew up with sadistic siblings know how unbearable being tickled can be, so it's no great surprise that a whole erotic tickling subculture exists. Unlike the wonderful world of pain, tickle torture is a bit deficient in the butch department; there's a big gap between a giggle and a groan. But, having been mercilessly tickled on occasion, I can attest that it is, in some ways, even worse than pain, a near-unbearable loss of control, hysterical laughter, gasping for breath. OK, I never found it particularly sexy, but when I discovered that Ticklefest, the annual convention of tickling fans, was due in San Francisco, it seemed like a worthy subject for, um, research.

I arrived at a local's apartment for the Ticklefest get-acquainted party to find about 30 men, an oddish bunch. The men grouped there seemed utterly average: some older, some younger, some cute, others handsome or craggy or just plain homely. The vibe, while friendly, was far from sex-drenched and not perceptibly kinky. Unlike the leather-and-pain shtick, tickling lacks semiotic-drenched clothing and props. There are feathers, but they seem a bit…ethereal. It seemed a lot like a foot-play crowd, nerdishness and all, and sure enough, one guy with a digital camera was wriggling around on the floor, taking shots of other men's bare feet.

The opening party was nice enough, in a wallflower-at-the-orgy way, but Ticklefest's main event was the next day's tickling marathon. Held at a local dungeon, the event was themed as a college frat initiation, with hazers and pledges identified by caps with, yes, feathers. The bottoms moved from one station to the next while sadistic tickling tops dug their fingers into foot soles, armpits, and tummies. It was contrived, and seemed to me as nonerotic as another man's fetish can get. Even the presence of good-looking bottoms and the chance to get my hands on those bottoms' feet and bellies didn't supersede the general geekiness of the scene. I could, intellectually, appreciate gasping outbreaks of helpless laughter, and I tried to put myself in a suitably sadistic mood. But not even the final farrago, when all the "frat brothers" tickled a pile of "pledges," seemed sexy. I suppose if I'd had an older butch brother who'd tickled me in childhood, it might have been otherwise. But I noticed that no one, neither ticklers nor ticklees, seemed to sport hard-ons. It was sex-as-pillowfight.

I left the party dissatisfied, feeling somewhat inadequate. I had to face it—I'd been bored. Alienated, even. Not at all tickled, pink or otherwise. I wasn't being judgmental, but somehow I felt that my empathy had failed. And I do so *want* to be cool.

Which is not to say that everyone has to find every kink stimulating. *There are plenty of things I get off on which other guys would look upon with a puzzled stare*, I told myself. *So I suppose that my sadism expressing itself as pleasantly moderate pain play is OK. I should stop being so hard on myself, huh?*

I did somewhat better at erotic wrestling.

My ball-torture friend Bret is into wrestling, the no-holds-barred version. Not quite wrestling-as-sex, more wrestling-as-aggression *followed* by sex. (Another friend, Jim, is part of a genuine, nonsexual gay wrestling league. He bristles when anyone suggests that all that grappling is just fucking in disguise. But that's another story.) As interested as I was in tough, hunky Bret and his matwork, he seemed a bit too much for me. So the idea that I might want to try a headlock or half nelson receded. But then I met Luke online. He liked to wrestle, naked, in his living room. We talked on the phone and made a date.

He's left his door open. I walk in and there he is, attractive, naked, and slim, with a dick that's attractive, naked, and fat. He's pushed back all the furniture. Two big futons cover most of the floor.

"You ready to wrestle for top, Daddy?" he taunts.

Well, uh, yes. I quickly strip down. We get face-to-face, real close, close enough for me to feel the heat of his cock. He sticks out a leg, grabs at me, and suddenly I'm flat on my back. With a hard-on. This is not, I realize, going to be as easy as I'd thought.

Luke is a lot smaller than me; I have 25 pounds and three or four inches on him. But he's in good shape, determined, experienced, and he is, after all, 15 years younger. And I haven't wrestled since high school, so I'm at something of a disadvantage. But as our nude, hairy bodies thrash around, hard-ons bobbing and weaving, I do my level best.

Well, sort of. We've agreed that our match was to be a struggle for domination: loser to be humiliated, face sat on, mouth fucked. Maybe he'll even get pissed on. But faced with a hunk like Luke, why *wouldn't* I want to lose and take my medicine? The temptation to throw the match is as great as if I'd laid big bucks on Luke at some Vegas sports book.

And so we go at it, around and around, him crushing my head between his thighs, me grabbing his balls and tugging, him slapping me, me punching him. "Dad," Luke grits out at one point, "you're a lot stronger than I'd thought." And suddenly all that time I'd spent at the Y doesn't seem like such a waste after all.

I strain mightily to show him who's boss, and he fights back with vigor, but every so often we just lie back exhausted and stroke each other sweatily. Eventually Luke does "overpower" me and shoves his butt against my face. I stick my tongue out and suffer mightily.

After some rimming and resting, it's time for a rematch. I manage to flip him down on his back and pin his wrists to the futon, er, mat, as we grind our hard dicks together. I kneel on his shoulders and "force" my cock into his mouth, the poor boy, while muttering whatever insults I still have enough breath left to hurl. Eventually it becomes quite clear that he doesn't really have to be forced to suck my cock, that in fact the line between winning and losing is thin and getting thinner all the time. But, as we lapse from hypermasculine struggle mode into homos having fun, we still punch each other every so often, just because.

Eventually, semi-exhausted, we jack each other off, taking charge of each other's cocks till they both shoot off, mixing cum with cum.

After wipe-up we sit around drinking green tea and chatting. Sweet guy. It turns out that his favorite author is, fairly improbably, Ralph Waldo Emerson. And a few days later, the few bruises will have faded, but my overworked triceps will still be a bit tender to the touch. Pleasant memories.

Control, it's so about control. Tied-up bottoms being flogged by their Masters. Men struggling naked for top. Sexual Holy Rollers speaking in tongues. (And I do wonder whether, when he's thrashing around on the floor of the local Pentecostal church, Joe Fundamentalist doesn't get an occasional hard-on.) Life is not a roller coaster, not really. It's a steep slide to oblivion, and only Hindus and Shirley MacLaine think that the re-rides are free. But we *like* roller coasters, don't we? There's the illusion that we're gonna—oh Christ, this first hill is really high—*die*. But we know the odds are we won't; otherwise, Six Flags would run out of customers pretty quick. We want to face oblivion, yeah, but we want to come back in one piece. It's just one of those weird things about human nature.

The French have nicknamed orgasm *le petit morte*, "the little death," and they certainly have a point. When pleasure and oblivion collide, it's a way powerful moment, so it's hardly a surprise that most of the world's great religions get so bent out of shape about lust and such. *Sin and salvation? Hey, that's OUR racket!*

If all sex is about loss of control, penetrating the boundaries of ego and flesh, then kink ups the ante. A lot of the safe-sane-and-consensual apologia for sadomasochistic fun skirt the issue, making a night in the dungeon sound as gosh-almighty good for you as aerobic step-dancing. And yes, in a funny way it is, but that's because kink is a dance through the sewer of life, a cha-cha in the gutter. Playing with pain is spitting in the face of Death.

How's *that* for pretension? I doubt even the French could do better.

CHAPTER 8
Welcome to the Woodshed: Punishment Scenes

Non-kinky people sometimes ask me, "So were you spanked as a child?" Though the answer is "No, not very much, not that I remember," I'm not sure why that's supposed to be relevant, anyway. After all, I was never sucked off as a child either, and now I like being blown just fine.

The very first kinky whatever I got into was indeed spanking. The specific memory is lost to me, but I know that somewhere along the line, maybe courtesy of an obliging trick, I realized that being spanked—and spanked fairly hard—felt real, real good. I don't know, maybe I even tried it out on myself first, in some sort of S/M masturbation. One 20-year-old I've met online does that sort of thing: He fantasizes being worked over, he approaches older men online and chats about over-the-knee butt beatings, but in real life he's a bit timid; the only hand that's ever whacked his butt is his own. Actually, he spanks himself quite a lot, which is rather innocent and sweet.

Swatting ass is one of the most popular bits of kink, which indicates it has a lot more going for it than a mere replaying of childhood trauma. Matter of fact, there are few bottoms I've played with who haven't responded cheerily to some sort of spanking, be it a few mild swats on the ass or a bottom-blistering assault that leaves their butt cheeks bright-red and hot as August.

Clearly, there's some hardwiring that makes getting spanked a joy. As many generations of sodomites can attest, our butt holes are rich in pleasure-producing nerves, ready to offer up bliss if we just relax and let 'em. Of all the places to enjoy the shifting borders between pleasure and pain, the ass is prime territory. Nicely padded, it lacks the "oh my God is this gonna harm me?" vulnerability of the dick and balls, but it's still a nice, juicy erogenous zone.

This boy who, years ago, accompanied me on some of my early steps down the Path to Perdition was into getting spanked. Big time. Big boy, actually. Taller than me, hopelessly boyish, with a lanky, smooth body that was still charmingly underdeveloped at 24. But a dick that was so adult-size it could take your breath away…in more ways than one. I first met Freddy on the phone sex lines; this was back in the pre-Internet era, somewhere between the Age of Steam and now. He had the sweetest little voice, almost childishly vulnerable, and our first conversation was immensely orgasmic. He couldn't give out his number—he was living with his boyfriend—but I gave him mine, and he phoned me again and again.

When we eventually met, I was bowled over. He was as innocent-looking as I'd hoped, as gawkily delightful as his voice had promised. Hell, he'd even decorated his bathroom in a *101 Dalmatians* motif. OK, he wasn't "handsome," was maybe not even "cute" in that way that perfect boys are cute. But God, he was sexy, and I really, really wanted him. He, though, was determined to honor his "monogamous" relationship, at least technically. There was a long list of things we couldn't do. But we could make out, we could strip down to our undies, I could even grope the rather enormous hard-on straining against his salmon-colored briefs.

And I could spank him.

If I wanted to.

I wanted to.

It was the first time I'd ever played with anyone so into having his ass worked over, and it was a revelation, though a short-lived one. Butting up against the borders of theoretical fidelity, he quickly called a halt to things, leaving me with blue balls and a smitten heart.

Freddy and I continued to play, oh, I don't know…cat and mouse? Boy and predator? Cocktease and teased? But over the months his relationship began breaking up, our meetings resumed, became more frequent, and we started having actual, cum-drenched sex.

This was back when I was just a semi-novice top. S/M folklore has it that all the good tops start as bottoms, and though I don't think that's necessarily the case, there's much to be said for the theory. I was once spanked by someone who was so incompetent, so totally lousy, that I was astonished. Spanking's not rocket science, not even close, and I know that anything erotic is a matter of taste, but still… That poor fellow, enthusiastic sadist though he may have been, was so clueless as to how to apply hand to butt that it was crushingly obvious that *he'd* never been spanked by someone who knew what they were doing. (Or if he had, he hadn't been paying attention.)

It became obvious, as I started going to play parties and meeting kinkier guys, that I, despite repeated readings of *The Leatherman's Handbook*, really didn't know what I was doing. So I started going to S/M classes.

There are, in San Francisco, a number of ways to learn the nuts and bolts of kink. There are gay men's discussion groups, all sorts of how-to sessions if you know where to find them. And there's a long-established school of S/M, I discovered, where folks of all genders and orientations matriculate in piss play and electrotorture. This was not in fact an actual school, with dormitories and a fight song and things; it was just a storefront where kinky people taught occasional classes in perversion. The place was run by Mistress Rita, a large, odd but personable Jewish-turned-Buddhist woman with an Ivy League education, a hankering for twisted sex, and a little brass school bell to signal the start of class.

After perusing one of her brochures, I'd arranged to help staff a class in return for free tuition. I suppose I'd hoped the classroom would be terribly atmospheric, but the place was a thoroughly utilitarian dive that, if stripped of its shelves of sex books, could have passed for an AA meeting place in a not very nice part of town. I set out the rows of folding chairs, stocked the concessions table with thawed frozen bagels and cans of Diet Coke, and waited for Abuse 101 to begin. And then Rita rang her bell.

I was eventually to take about a dozen classes at Mistress Rita's place. (It was where I took those bondage lessons too.) The classes were largely straight-oriented, attended by mostly attractive women and mostly dweeby men; I was often the only queer man in attendance. No matter; I was eager to learn the fine art of working over the human body. Kind of geeky? Well, who but kinky nerds would pay good money to sit on folding chairs and take notes on cock torture? At Mistress Rita's I learned how to paddle, flog, and encourage a bottom to process pain cheerfully. I watched a bear get play-pierced with a couple of dozen needles, a woman in puffy pants pretending to be another woman's harem slave, and a guy sticking a dildo up his girlfriend's butt. I took part in a discussion of the modalities of verbal abuse, and I watched a suspension scene in which a tied-up naked guy dangled from hooks in the ceiling. It was, indeed, quite an education. Finally, though, I got bored with tallying book sales, selling packaged brownies, and—worst of all for a not very submissive guy

like me—vacuuming Rita's room and making her always messy
bed. Still, I got a chance to watch some of the kinkiest folks in
town in action. (It's where I first met Carol Queen, who's one of
this country's foremost campaigners for more and better sex. I
can't imagine a perkier, more ingratiating teacher of piss play.)

I learned lots of useful stuff at those classes. I learned that not
every woman into kink looks like the high-cheekboned models
wearing thigh-high boots in *Skin Two* magazine. Some, in fact,
look like your mother. On a bad day. I learned that there is no
final arbiter of the right way to tie someone up, or the right way
to slap someone around, or the right way to fuck. And I learned
that, as someone said, "One man's eroticism is another man's
belly laugh." I can still see myself there, all eager to learn, perched
on an uncomfortable chair, as several feet away people were
doing unspeakable things to one another while I took copious
notes. Ah, alma mater.

What I did not get from the class was laid. Fortunately, by that
time I'd found Freddy to do my homework on. Despite a last-
ditch effort to save their relationship by buying a black BMW
together, Freddy and his boyfriend had called it quits. The field
was clear. And I made the most of it. I was, I now realize, greedy.
Greedy for what I'd never had before—a cute young fellow who'd
let me do simply awful things to his naked body. I suppose the
Buddha could have maintained a modicum of detachment under
these circumstances, but I sure as hell couldn't. I practiced my
bondage moves on him, we explored daddy/boy play, but most of
all, I spanked his butt.

I spanked him with his pants on, I spanked him through his
briefs, I spanked him on his perfect, smooth, bare ass. I spanked
him till he squirmed, till he tried to get away, sometimes till he
started sobbing. And he loved every damn near-unbearable
minute.

We started going to dungeon parties together. He'd never played in public before, and I found his virginal nervousness a total aphrodisiac. When I first locked him into stocks, he shook so hard that everything rattled. This charmed the onlookers, and I could have, as my grandmother would have said, *plotst*. We became quite a team. I'd lead him by a leash through one dungeon or another, tie him down, and proceed to alternately spank him and stroke him till he reached the lovely, dark place we both were aiming for. We sometimes gathered quite a crowd; the spectacle of lean, smooth Freddy roped facedown to a bondage table, trembling there with a beautiful, bright-red ass, sure was worth a look.

We also—and here I can sort of see what might have gone wrong—became friends. Good friends. Now, in the best of all possible worlds, fuck buddies, especially cute, masochistic fuck buddies with *101 Dalmatians* shower curtains, *would* become your friends, right? Why separate sex and affection? Isn't that armored and instrumentalist and, um, dysfunctional? Well, sure, but…if you're some boy in his early 20s who is still finding your feet, socially speaking, and you find yourself going to the beach and the ballet with a man twice your age, a man who on a regular basis strips you down, dominates you, and inflicts erotic pain, mightn't it get a bit…confusing? Well, sure. Especially when the older man has a crush on you, as I undeniably did on young Freddy.

And there was one other thing about Freddy: He wouldn't kiss. It wasn't a butch thing, because heaven knows, he was far from macho. It was a disease thing, a fear of HIV, or so he said. Oh, he would dry-kiss, a little puckered-up brush against my lips. But for someone who was otherwise so wide-open to all sorts of stuff, the no-kiss rule was bothersome. Sure, he was, strictly speaking, right, since kissing can transmit diseases (though not HIV), but his reticence eventually took on symbolic significance for me. All that kink, those extreme states of being, that sexual intimacy, and then…no tangling of tongues and swapping of spit? It was as if kissing would make us seem like boyfriends. And Freddy was having none of that.

My up-and-down relationship with Freddy lasted the better part of four years. Eventually he moved to the suburbs with his new (and dismayingly vanilla) boyfriend, but by then he'd hardly ever return my phone messages. Finally he confessed that he'd found another Daddy, a retiree with a bad ticker and money to burn. Dad bought Freddy a swank black leather jacket, took him on trips to Vegas, and eventually dropped dead of cardiac arrest.

Shortly thereafter, Freddy and his boyfriend broke up; their buying a house together had apparently been as inauspicious a move as the purchase of the black Beemer in his previous relationship. Freddy thereafter moved back to Arizona, where he continued to play with one of the West's most notoriously expert spankers. I was tooling around the Web when I found the spanker's site, which prominently featured photos of young, virginal, reticent Freddy, usually buck naked, though in one delightfully sick picture he was wearing a Cub Scout uniform. I was either pleased or distressed to note that he'd apparently put on weight and would with any luck be portly by the time he reached middle age. In one series of shots he and another fellow—younger, skinnier, more classically cute—were romping around the desert, their butts freshly spanked, and in one shot they were kissing.

Wet-kissing.

After Freddy and his beautiful butt, there came a procession of asses to be abused. White asses, black asses, yellow, and brown; hairy, smooth, big or skinny; young or not so. I've spanked them all, and, if I may be permitted a moment of pride, I think I spanked them rather well. I've used a leather paddle, a hairbrush, a strap, a wooden paddle, a riding crop, a variety of floggers, a bamboo switch, a fiberglass cane, and a leather-covered hitting stick that I think of as, imaginatively, "the leather-covered hitting stick," but somehow I still like using my bare hand most of all. The intimacy of flesh hitting naked, vulnerable flesh; the ease of switching from spanking to stroking and back again; the basic, old-fashioned nature of bare hand–to–bare bottom spanking— all work really well for me.

And then there are the psychological overtones of the sport. In civilian life spanking remains, after all, a punishment doled out to a naughty child. There are some adult kinksters who like to play spanking strictly as a punishment scene too, but that's precisely where things get murky. In a consensual scene, of course, getting spanked is just what the bottom *craves*, and there's a certain ambiguity in situations where "punishment" and pleasure are one and the same. For the longest time I—who knows full well the joys of getting one's ass whupped—found the desire of some bottoms to frame spanking scenes as punishment to be transparent and rather silly. Then I began to ask myself just what they were being punished *for*. Skipping school? Breaking Mom's good china? Unlikely. They were, I realized, being punished precisely for the desire to get spanked: i.e., for being big faggot perverts. Just as, in a Buddhist sense, the journey and the goal are one, when it comes to discipline scenes the transgression and the punishment are one. I find this thoroughly marvelous, genuine Instant Karma, a Zen koan of pain and need. It's the old yin-yang thing, with a flogger in its hand.

This *can* stretch the boundaries of credulity. Remember, the top—a.k.a. the dominant or "dom"—who's doing the "disciplin-ing" is expected to act as though he's "forcing" the other guy into something which is, after all, profoundly desired. And the putative submissive, or "sub," gets just exactly what he wants. This "let's pretend" aspect of punishment scenes is one reason they've never particularly appealed to me; if there's going to be suffering in a scene, I'd rather it start out from a more real place. Still, many bottoms do want to be punished for something, anything. It is, I suppose, a working through of various guilts which, when it comes to sexual desire, are usually over things no one should feel guilty about to start with.

And that brings up homophobia. While I'm sure straight guys being worked over by female dommes do have their own sets of things to feel regret for—hetero hegemony, an unwillingness to reciprocate during oral sex, the Republican Party—their kinkiest lusts are just variations on mandatory heterosexuality. I'd guess, based on precisely no empirical evidence, that gay punishment scenes cut a lot deeper than similar het play, since a queer bottom not only gets to feel guilty about his variant desires but his most basic ground of being. Which may (or may not) be one reason S/M seems to be more widely practiced, accepted, even valorized in the queer world than in its breeder counterpart. We've failed our parents, our world, maybe even ourselves, and we deserved to get spanked. Damn it, we *do*.

And the top? He gets the chance to play angry parent, to be on the other side of condemnation, for once. To transcend faghood and be bad-ass as any straight dude.

Hold still, you little cocksucker, while Daddy tans your evil hide. You little sissyfuck, how dare you make me do this to you? You know I fucking love you. I'm only doing this for your own good. And it hurts me more than it hurts you. Or maybe, just maybe, it—heh heh—DOESN'T! Whack. Whack, whack, whack.

So, yes, some of the erotic charge of spanking goes back to childhood, whether or not we were actually spanked as kids, whether our parents were straitlaced, condemnatory Baptists, or sweet-tempered PFLAG folks who encouraged you to have your boyfriend sleep over. It's the kind of universal expiation for sin that's Christianity's stock-in-trade, which probably explains all those medieval monks running around flogging themselves.

One of the nicest things about kink is that, despite the smiley-face hype of its cheerier proponents, it isn't a solution to *anything*—just a series of questions, thornier and thornier, darker and darker, stretching from the soul all the way to the horizon. And one of the many puzzles is whether this sort of play is therapeutic, allowing us to work through inner conflicts in a safe, eroticized, circumscribed field of action, or just a fucked-up, compulsive, neurotic replay of some really sick shit.

This particular conundrum hit me full force several years back. I'd met a handsome butch man in his late 30s, an accomplished queer performing artist, well-known on the national scene, who was visiting from the East Coast. I was in fact a bit in awe of the guy, and when I met him I felt like something of a groupie. There was, it turned out, some sexual heat there, and our brief meeting turned into an all-night discussion.

Jack was, beneath his craggily good-looking face and quiet masculinity, something of a masochist. And, it turned out, he really *had* been abused as a child. His stepfather had beaten him, frequently and mercilessly. As he told the story of his childhood, probably for the thousandth time, there was a look of genuine pain on his sexy face. I had the feeling of being let in to view forbidden territory, and, as it often does in similar circumstances, this feeling resulted in a hard-on that just wouldn't quit.

We ended up making a date for the next evening. Throughout the day I couldn't get him out of my mind, and when I showed up at his hotel room I was faint with anticipation and desire. We kissed and caressed and then, as had been previously discussed, my caresses turned into something altogether rougher. I tore off his shirt, buttons popping everywhere, and started slapping his naked chest.

He was fully erect, totally lost in lust, and I was absolutely turned on. When I'd stripped him down to his briefs, precum seeping through the cotton, I shoved him down on the bed and started hitting him for real.

"You can punch me in my gut," he gasped. "I'd like that"—a pause—"Daddy."

And as I slugged him—not pausing for my usual stroking and kissing, just pounding away, watching his semi-famous face writhe in ecstasies of pain—I began to feel uneasy. Not uneasy enough to stop, not nearly. But there I was rummaging around a broken soul so injured, so wide-open; the responsibility—no matter how often he'd done this scene, with however many men—felt awesome. We're all so injured, with so much longing, so much pain, and here was this man, a near-stranger, smart and beautiful, suddenly becoming a scared, love-hungry little boy when I put my boot in.

I'm a careful, conscious top. I'd never cause intentional, real harm. But as this scene spiraled upward, my inner sadist took wing.

"You fucking *boy*. Fucking boy fucking boy fucking boy." The asshole had forced me to be evil, and he was going to pay for that. But I was, I'll bet, a lot more scared than he was about what was going on. I tore off his briefs and went to work on his naked ass, slapping his hard dick around, punching and kicking. Doing it carefully, but punching and kicking and slapping him and suddenly seeing all of human possibility stretched out before me in a dark, dark glory of mortality, memory, and love.

"You COCKSUCKING SON OF A FAGGOT BITCH!"

There were tears in his eyes.

"Oh Daddy Daddy Daddy," he moaned from between clenched teeth. He'd become the little boy, the scared little boy he'd once been for real, quivering before the angry power of his abusive stepfather. It was there. It was all right there, and despite all the contrivances, it was real and it was true.

And then he came. It wasn't an ejaculation, not really; it was a slow oozing and flowing, a flood of thick, yellowish cum, and as I reached down, jacked off, and shot a load all over his beautiful body, all over his damaged soul, I was shaking, and not just from the orgasm. I was thoroughly shook.

Only then did I stroke him, kiss him, and wipe his tender boytears away.

"I usually don't go that deep with guys," he said. I didn't know if that was true, but I wanted to believe it, so I did.

We lay together, sticky and panting, for a while. There was a lot I wanted to to say, to ask, but despite what had just happened, our intimacy had its limits. Eventually we drifted off to small talk, I got dressed, and lacking an invitation to stay the night, an invitation I craved, I headed for home.

Years later I sometimes see his face in the media, and I remember that scene more vividly than last week's trick. He did return to San Francisco, I left a message for him, but he never got back to me. It's probably just as well. Some things have their natural arcs that would be ruined by trying for more.

But that radical vulnerability of his still haunts me. What, just exactly what, happened that night at his hotel? Was it the blossoming of some strange beauty—a reconciliation of the hopelessly damaged past and the hopeful, erotic present? Was it, truly, therapy for lost dreams? Or was it just a driven, neurotic replay of scripts that should have been burned years ago? More harm than good? Might I have even, not with my fists but in some more profound way, done damage? Was I even, in some way that theology can't quite touch, truly evil?

Well, who the fuck knows? It would take a lifetime, maybe many lifetimes, to answer those questions, to soothe those aching chunks of karma.

All I know is that Madonna can warble smarmily about a bit of spanky-panky, countless sitcoms can make jokes about erotic butt beatings, but what lies beneath, what can sometimes be reached not just as theater, not merely as a playroom scene, but for one darkly glowing instant can actually be experienced, *that's* what's real. Or as real as anything can be in this world of *maya*, of illusions that pose as truth.

All it takes is a wave of the hand.

CHAPTER 9
This Way to the Ninth Circle: S/M Play Parties

I'm at an S/M sex party when I run into my friend Dave, a hunky bisexual with a great chest that he never hesitates, not the slightest bit, to display. He's been involved, he tells me, in the shooting of a how-to S/M video. The star of the show, a professional dominatrix with even bigger tits than Dave's, has spared no expense, hiring a professional videographer and making sure the lighting, makeup and costumes are first-rate. Dave is proud to be part of such a top-of-the-line production, and I can't say I blame him, but I'm in a semi-evil mood, so I say, "Well, that's what all of this S/M stuff is all about, right? Show business?"

And he, like an eager irony-free puppy, nods his head in agreement.

Show business.

When I first started going to dungeon parties, I was totally awestruck and more than a little excited. Amazing: Here were all these more-or-less naked people doing all these perfectly horrid things to one another and, for the price of admission, I could watch. Maybe even—someday—join in.

It's like walking into one of those movies about the decadence of Weimar Berlin. You stroll into the play space, hand over your invitation and the entrance fee. There's a changing room filled with men stripping off street clothes, then putting on leather chaps and harnesses, cock rings and ball stretchers, as well as other, weirder fetish gear. Some of them are wearing whole leather stores on their backs—for what they've paid for their shiny, studded togs, you could feed a Third World village for a year. They dress up as fantasies: their own or what they assume are the fantasies of the guys they'd like to play with. And some of them do indeed look astonishingly hot. Astonishingly.

Then it's down a corridor or through a door, sometimes down dimly lit stairs, to the dungeon. Even before your eyes adjust to the semi-gloom, you can hear what's happening: floggers, whips, and paddles meeting flesh; the moans of tied-up men. And then it comes into view: a room chock-full of hardcore perversion at its best. Men tied to hooks in the walls or to bondage tables, men with electrified butt plugs up their asses, men being pierced with dozens of hypodermic points, men being whipped till their backs bleed. And then some. Welcome to the theme park from hell.

So what's a nice boy like you doing in a place like this?

Oddly enough, considering I'm such a total fag, the first parties I ever went to were mixed—men, women, gay, straight, bi. So there I was, still in the embryonic phase of kinkhood, watching leatherdykes carving Celtic designs into one another's shoulders to the music of thudding floggers and moaning bottomgirls. Fortunately, there were also enough gay guys there to make me feel like I could score, and enough willing ones so that I *did* score, at least every once in a while.

When I first started playing at parties, I was like a kid in a very twisted candy store. Suddenly I was doing things I'd only dreamed about, and more than a few things that I'd never even considered. Suddenly, I was spanking Dino—a cute little Italian bi guy with a *very* spankable cute little ass—in public. He was affectionate, friendly, and obligingly let me work him over whenever he wasn't otherwise engaged.

And was that really little ol' me tying Len's wrists to a hook in the ceiling—his lean, hairy body stretched to its limits, his hard-on standing straight up, eager for abuse? Gee willikers, this was fun!

Things got even hotter when I started playing with my fuck buddy Freddy. As we continued to play, in private and public, over many months we honed our act so that when I'd tie him up and slap him around at a party we'd usually gather an appreciative audience. It was hot to be admired for my rope work; it was great when our play excited other men and they stood there jacking off. Now, in some sense, all sex is performance, but being onstage in the dungeon was new to me. Guys were actually coming up and asking to bottom for me, and any top knows what a rush that can be.

The more Freddy and I played in public, the hotter it got. We became seasoned troupers, able to get into the swing of things and give, dare I say it, a really good show.

However it may look from the outside, a good dungeon scene is a collaboration, a delicate tango of meshing needs and desires. It's not a free-for-all with whips. One of the good things about invitation-only S/M parties is that you end up with a group of guys who are experienced, respectful, and smart. It wasn't till I played at a sex club open to the general public that I grasped the differences. A good public scene is prenegotiated, or at least not up for grabs; anyone with an iota of experience knows that there are protocols to be followed. But when I took one ultra-cute boy to a mega–sex club, a place open to anyone with a dick and 10 bucks, and tied him to the bars of a jail cell in the "cellblock," civilian passersby acted as though I was just giving him away. Without hesitation, the rank amateurs just moved right in for a piece of the meat, not understanding (or caring) that I was not just in control of the scene but responsible for the well-being of my bottomboy too. The sub, kinky as he was, didn't really want to be pawed over by all and sundry, so I spent half my time keeping horny buggers with wandering hands from horning in. Tedious.

Often, when novices ask me about play parties, the number one question is, "Do I have to do anything, or can I just stand there and watch?" I've never been to a party where observers, at least observers who kept a respectful distance and didn't chatter like tweaked Chihuahuas, were unwelcome. Because S/M play parties *are* showbiz, partly. Everybody's up on stage, doing their schtick in full view of everyone else, and all but the shyest actors crave an appreciative audience. Still, just standing there watching is like going to the Castro District on Halloween without a costume. You can look around, ogle, and goggle without putting anything at risk. It's a tourist position, and it can be fun, but it's no match for dressing up, slipping on a mask, and letting yourself be someone else for the night. Going to a play party just to watch can be enjoyable, in a voyeuristic kind of way. But there's something of the wallflower about it. *Here I am, all dressed up, and nobody's asked me to dance.*

I'm at the same old S/M party again, watching Paco, the Michelangelo of play-piercing, once again doing a masterful scene. There is, cutely, a little headlamp strapped to his forehead so he can see what he's doing in the gloom; he looks like he's mining for masochists. A 60-ish gent covered from collarbone to foot with Maori tattoos lies squirming as my pal pins down his dick and balls, which protrude through a hole in a little board laid on his crotch. As needle after needle fastens his delicate parts to the board, what had been his genitals begin to look like a planked fish in a tony French cookbook. His face, though, is somewhere east of ecstasy, and every time a needle slides through scrotal flesh, his body gives a satisfying little jerk.

Nearby, three guys who look like nice, vanilla fagboys dipping their toes into the swamp of kink gawk and giggle. One of them, the blond, is cute enough to slap around hard. *I'll wipe that smirk off your face, sonny boy!*

Harold, meanwhile, has two bottomboys facedown, side by side, arms around one another as he beats the hell out of their adjoining asses. And on the other side of the room, a man (who I might have recognized had his head not been enclosed in a leather hood) is busy shooting sperm as electrodes send jolts of voltage through his dick. I feel both like I'm part of the scene, an experienced player who's welcome at the orgy, and on the other hand like an alienated outsider shut off from the hearty camaraderie of the whippers and the just-whipped. I think back to my conversation with Dave some weeks earlier: It all *does* seem like showbiz.

I'm just about to chuck it and head for home when I hear cries from the adjoining room, the smaller space with the cages and the rack. There's a man wearing only chaps, tied facedown to the rack. A top perhaps 10 years older, mid 40s, is working him over, using a lightweight flogger and a small paddle, nothing heavy-duty. But the bottom is crying out and squirming with every stroke.

"Let it out, Steve, let it go," the top urges. "Give it to me, Steve."

Steve is clearly teetering on the brink of his limits. He's apparently been tenderized, so even a small stroke sends intense sensation through his already sensitized flesh. He's on the verge of tears. He has a runny nose. And all this gets my dick hard, instantly. Clearly, something *real* is at stake.

"I can't take it, Sir. I can't take anymore."

"Sure you can, Steve," urges the topman, gently but firmly, or at least as gently as a man with a flogger can. He's playing his bottomboy like a violin with balls. Impressed, I'm wishing I were him, able to guide Steve through this very public ritual. But then, part of me is wishing I were Steve, suffering under the whip hand of such a caring top.

"No!" screams Steve as the back of his thighs gets swacked.

"Don't say 'no,' Steve. Say 'yes.' " And another blow.

"Yes," groans Steve from between gritted teeth. "Yesyesyes."

Real vulnerability, the kind that can't be readily faked, radiates from the tied-down man with the reddened ass. I'm thoroughly hypnotized by the scene, a cobra who has spotted his prey through a windowpane, so tempting yet inaccessible.

"Let it out, Steve. Let it out."

There's a code of behavior at play parties, and every player worth his cock ring respects it. I could walk over, say respectfully to the top, "Nice scene, good bottomboy. Mind if I join in?" Part of me wants to—badly. But there's something about this particular interchange, this dance of will and flesh, that seems…well, *sacred* sounds pretentious, but it's not too strong a word.

I realize that not everyone is as fascinated by this scene as I am. Guys wander by, watch for a minute or two, then walk on. Paco's play-piercing, with its showy geometries of hypodermic points patterning his bottom's naked torso, has gathered a bigger audience. The needlework is gorgeous, true, but over at the rack things are deep and real: the kind of moment that can only be reached, I'm thinking, by a collaboration of men in sync, men who trust each other—a top who knows just what to do, a bottom willing to go into his own private darkness. I know the feelings firsthand. I've been there, sometimes as a top, more rarely as a bottom. It's the heartbreakingly elusive possibility in S/M, as in all extreme yogas, of some sort of sought transcendence—of, as Leonard Cohen sings, "the card so high and wild he'll never need to deal another." But this sort of chemistry isn't all that common, and I am enthralled by its unfolding. Jesus, is my dick hard.

"Say it, Steve. Say the word."

"I don't know what the word *is*, Sir. I don't know the fucking word."

I assume this is about safewords. The top was saying, *You know how to make this end. Say the safeword and I'll stop—this will all be over.* And the bottom replied, *Part of me wants to use the safeword, part of me hurts too much, doesn't know how much more I can take, but another part of me wants this never, ever to end, and where's that at?*

And then the scene does end. Steve has taken all he could take, his top has dished out all he's going to inflict. Everything starts floating down to Earth, sparks stop shooting around the room. I want to go over, tell the two of them how much their scene has meant to me. But Steve, released from the clutches of the rack, has been enfolded in the older, bigger man's arms, is being stroked and cajoled back to tranquility. It's a private moment in a public space, and I wander off, hesitant to intrude.

It's only when the long-lasting hug has ended and the two are gathering up the ropes and restraints that I approach them. "You're amazing," I say to the top, who makes suitably modest noises, and to Steve I say, "You're a very lucky boy."

Perhaps 20 minutes later, I'm in the kitchen upstairs, nibbling on a cookie that really isn't very good for me. Steve comes in.

"How you doing?" I say, thinking maybe he'd want to play with me sometime.

"He's waiting for me, I've gotta get going," Steve says.

"Great scene."

"Really?"

"Yeah," I say. "How long have you two been playing?"

"We just met tonight," Steve says glumly, "and I feel like I let him down. I feel like a total wimp."

I do a double take. I want to drag out my usual line: *Well, it's not a contest, you know.* But I wasn't sure he *did* know.

"I've never done that before," Steve says. Which shows me how off-base I could be. Steve isn't being disingenuous. He really does think the scene was a flop, that he was disappointing. I wonder how the top feels about it. Well, they *are* leaving together.

And Steve shuffles out of the room.

Later I'll tell my friend Bull, a Buddhist of the stoned S/M variety, about this story. "Was I wrong about what was happening in that scene?" I'll ask. "Was I just seeing what I wanted to see?"

"I wouldn't take what Steve said too seriously," Bull will reply. "It may take him 10 years to figure out what happened tonight."

Ten years.

Sadomasochistic sex, especially the traditional leathersex variety, is chockablock with rules and rituals. It's fun, of course, in the way that being initiated into the Masons must be fun. But these road rules also exist because this stuff is scary. The clubby aspects of "the leather community" paper over some less-than-simple realities. Let's face it, there's something dark and disturbing about the notion of going into a roomful of strangers, stripping your clothes off, being tied down, and getting whipped till you cry. Not that this sort of thing is "bad," necessarily, much less utterly evil. But it's not the same as a bingo game. Kink involves a radical vulnerability that is always at least a little risky. It's letting the big, hungry animal out to play.

Dungeon parties provide a safe space to do that. It's public play, so things can't get seriously out of hand; the dungeon master, a twisted chaperone wearing an armband or special cap, sees to that. Usually the rules are posted and clear, and you have to agree to them in writing. Some of the rules are about safety:

gloves for fisting, rubbers for fucking, limits to be respected. Others are Miss Manners for masochists: Don't horn in on a scene, don't distract players with loud talk. Some parties—rather pissily—dictate style: no street clothes, or maybe no running shoes. And never, ever wear cologne.

Down in the dungeon you're surrounded by like-minded men, so no one will look askance if you get a hard-on from being hit on your bare bottom. What's more, there's an available cast of potential playmates; with a bit of spontaneity, two-person scenes can turn into interesting orgies. There's plenty of room to use elaborate equipment, swing a whip, escape the boyfriend. There are aspects of public play—exhibitionism, public humiliation—that can't be easily reproduced at home. And it's a dandy place to meet guys who're into what you're into, from fisting to feet.

Why, then, have play parties lost some of their luster for me? Part of it is the clubbiness. The notion of "the leather communi-ty" is a slippery one, but there are certainly social ties among leathermen. Sometimes at play parties there are more men on the patio snacking, smoking, and gossiping than there are down in the dungeon. It's like an uneasy cross between the decadent depths of Weimar Berlin and a Rotarians meeting. Newly whipped boys compare their welts, evil pervs chat about their Web sites, sadists trade tech tips on electro-torture. For a while, before the dot-com crash, there was much talk of portfolios. And let's face it, you haven't lived till you've heard a bunch of beard-ed men with whips sitting around discussing Cher's farewell concert. It's all very gemütlich.

And yet, and yet…that old black magic can in fact happen. I can be swept away by a scene, a new partner, a situation that makes both my dick and my brain lose their critical distance. At that play party, after Steve and his new Master have left the build-ing, I wander off to the social room. A guy I've seen all night, great-looking, naked except for a baseball cap, seemingly self-absorbed, almost always jacking off, always avoiding my eye, is sprawled on the sofa, naked, legs spread. I figure that Jack-off Boy has been avoiding me because I'm insufficiently Adonislike, but my friend Paco is kneeling between the boy's spread legs, and Paco, for all his sterling traits and piercing skills, is hardly a conventional hunk. Jack-off Boy is still engaged in self-abuse, but now his family jewels are in Paco's firm grasp, and Paco is pulling, twisting, and slapping while the naked boy on the sofa writhes and moans. I smile at Paco, and he smiles back with a "come and join me" grin. I sidle up to the boy, and Jack-off Boy smiles too, and nods. My ego zooms from zero to 60 in five seconds flat. There I am, playing with one of the hottest guys at the party, slapping his firm, inviting inner thighs and nipping at his tits. Turns out that Paco has to head for home, and he's leaving the boy in my I-hope-capable hands.

I decide it's time to introduce myself. His name is Scott, and he tells me that he's pretty much a novice—this is his first time at a leather-sex party. But he's often fantasized about being tied down firmly and milked of his cum, and did I think I might be into doing that?

I say a silent *thank you* to the gods of perversion and lead Scott down to the dungeon. He's already stripped down, of course, so I pull my restraints and ropes out of my toy bag and get down to work. Scott lies there, pulling on his well-used dick, applying frequent gobs of lube. *Even with the lube*, I think, *that pretty thing is going to be blistered in the morning.*

It's been awhile since I tied up anyone in public, and I'm thoroughly enjoying myself. I wrap ropes around his legs, working from the ankles upward, till his thighs are restrained by a network of ropes anchored to the webbing of the rack. As I go to work on tying down his torso, I notice from the corner of my eye that a couple of guys are watching us. Knowing I'm working for an audience, I try to make every move as Masterful as possible, every rope taut, every knot perfectly achieved. I confess—I'm a ham.

When it's time to restrain Scott's arms and hands, he asks, "You'll jack me off while I'm tied down, right?"

"Yeah," I attempt to growl. "Didn't I tell you that I would?"

Like there's a chance in hell I won't.

For all the planning that can go into a scene, there's something about surprises. Surprises like Scott. One of the delightful things about dungeon parties is the opportunity to get into scenes you otherwise might have missed out on. Wondering about how it feels to be play-pierced? To be hung from the ceiling? To endure the pain of a single-tail whip? With diplomacy, tact, and a dab of luck, play parties give you a chance to find out. (And take it from me, that single-tail whip hurts like a motherfucker.)

At parties you get to play with men you otherwise might never have met, at least not in the nude. I've found myself in a bondage four-way, two of us tops tying two bottomboys together. There was that bondage-bag scene where five or six of us worked over a lucky guy totally encased in pricey black leather, a bit of kit beyond the means of most freelance porn writers.

And then there was the evening I spent with the duo of thoroughly wired speed freaks, cutely disreputable-looking boys. One was paddling the other, rather disconsolately, when I came over to watch. I had my flogger in hand.

"Maybe you want to take a turn with him?" the "top" said after a while.

I looked at the bottomboy, who radiated "street trash"—the baggy pants that were the current mode; shaggy, unwashed hair; tough little face; shirtless torso decorated with a few really lousy tattoos, the handmade kind you get when you're drunk or in jail. The kind of lad, in other words, whom I'd probably never meet—not on the street, not even in a bar, and definitely the kind of boy I wouldn't drag home to my place and allow into my apartment, not even if I were stoned and desperate. So would I top the little piece of rough trade? Shit yeah.

The kid responded well to my flogging. He wasn't much for pain, but he was fun. Good, dirty fun. With a woody.

I'm not the sort of guy who thrives on rough trade, not really. I don't fetishize seeming straightness, and my self-destructive tendencies are channeled in ways unlikely to leave me tied up and beaten by a guy who looks like he just escaped from the slammer. But I understand, I think, why some guys thrive on that sort of danger. It must have something to do with the urge to punish ourselves for our perverted desires. Those into rough trade seek out these icons of hypermasculinity not only because they're butch—it's because they're the kind of "butch" likely to beat up the faggots who find them so attractive.

This bottomboy, anyway, seemed less the type who'd assault you for your wallet than the sort of boy who'd sneak out with your CD collection while you were in the bathroom. He was, in his very wired way, kind of sweet. When he dropped his saggy trousers so I could work over his butt, he turned out to be kind of smelly too. I only hoped that if he had scabies, they'd unadventurously stay home on him.

The boy would, I'd correctly figured, be the no-kissing type. But rather surprisingly, he wouldn't let me suck his fat uncut cock either. Rough trade, of course, is supposed to be serviced—that's their role in life—but in hygienic retrospect I suppose it was just as well. Actually, I wish I'd told his friend to suck his dick while I beat the shit out of both of them, but hindsight is 20/20.

As it happened, the bottomboy came while I slapped him

around, his friend jacked off while watching, and that was pretty much that. A bit of conversation elicited the fact that the only reason they were at the party was that they were crashing with one of the older guys there—a man who, I knew, had a rather unsavory reputation where young men, drugs, and sex were concerned.

I went upstairs to take a break from the tag-team speed freaks. Bull was there.

"You looked like you were having fun down there," he smiled.

"Yeah," I said, stuffing yet another disastrously high-fat cookie in my mouth.

"You really like boys who are trouble," Bull said.

"You know me too well."

"I just hope," he said, "you didn't give them your phone number."

Some of what happens at play parties is impossible to reproduce at home. There's the opportunity to watch some truly amazing men doing truly astonishing stuff. There are the chance meetings, the possibility of meeting Master Right or the perfect boy, not to mention having enough room to swing a cat-o'-nine-tails, play space being at a premium in the always overpriced San Francisco housing market. The equipment in a well-furnished dungeon—stocks, St. Andrew's cross, cages, slings, and racks—allow a range of play scenes far beyond the horizons of the average bedroom. But perhaps most crucially, there's the chance to feel like you *belong*, that you're part of a semisecret society with its own uniforms and rituals. Almost despite itself, the world of gay S/M has created new, and real, sorts of communities. And there's no doubt that, despite what may look to jaundiced eyes like half-assed ass whuppings and overscripted scenes, many men have gone through some pretty profound stuff on their way between the check-in desk and a post-abuse can of Pepsi.

AIDS pretty much decimated a whole generation of hard-core leathermen, and the monthly parties I go to, whatever else they might be, are also gatherings of what's left of the tribe. They're an opportunity to learn the folkways, to find an experienced top to put you through your paces or a willing bottom to try stuff out on, all within a safe, monitored environment. And they provide reassurance that perversion—like Gloria Gaynor—will survive.

On some nights, parties can seem as dull to me as the worst night in a vanilla gay bar; on others, pure lunatic magic. It's a matter of chance, to some extent: who's playing, which scenes manage to reach critical mass. But, like life itself, it's also a matter of subjectivity, of what a guest brings to the party.

I'm at the same old dungeon, the same old guys doing the same old things, and I'm utterly disengaged. Yes, Harold is paddling a boy I wish I were working over; and yes, Paco's play-piercing scene is gorgeous as usual; and there's a beautiful guy I've never seen wandering around naked, his hands tied behind his back, clamps on his nipples; but I'm in a played-out mode, having worked over a delightfully greedy Nik earlier that day, and don't score high enough on the hornymeter to risk rejection. Here I am afloat in a stew pot of hard-core lust, and I'm bored bored bored.

And that's when I see him: 30-ish, fully dressed (though not in leather), cute, with long, dark hair hanging all the way down his back, all the way to his butt. He is, I figure, a shade out of my league, though he's just standing around, checking out the scenes. Maybe his un-modish hair and non-reg outfit are hurting his chances. But hey, I'd fuck him, no problem.

I try catching his eye but get nothing beyond a noncommittal nod my way. So I sigh silently and go upstairs to get a beer. I'm just sitting around, watching a video of a few shaved boys desultorily pretending to get off on spanking each other, when the longhair guy appears, a little plate of chips and dip in one hand. Snacks. (What's odd about dungeon parties, at least most of the ones I've been to, is that they tread on such potentially frightening ground, but they seem so damn *normal*, as if there's nothing strange about discussing the opera season while just yards away some fellow is being tortured with hot wax.)

So, gathering up the last shreds of inertial courage, I walk over to him and say, stupidly I suppose, "How's it going?" In a matter of minutes we're down in the dungeon again. He's naked, on all fours, long hair everywhere, sucking my cock as I slide my gloved hand up past his well-trained sphincter. Suddenly, like a wallflower being asked to dance, I am transformed. I'm part of the fun, part of the flow, and what had seemed like a dreary retread of parties past is now a shining vortex of lust. And when I finally cum, I cum long, hard, and copiously.

Reeking of male sweat, poppers, and cum, the dungeon is no doubt a place that would scare some folks out of their skins. To others of us, though, it's a place of bonding, of discovery, and reassuring—if theatrical—fun.

It's quite a club. If only it didn't seem, sometimes, quite so much like the Rotarians.

CHAPTER 10
Doing It in the Road:
Street Fairs and Shamelessness

The day of the Folsom Street Fair dawns, as many September days in San Francisco do, warm and piercingly blue. I pull on my well-worn chaps and head out the door, not so much because I really want to go as because I'm afraid that if I stay home with the Sunday *Chronicle*, I'll miss something.

As I ride my motorcycle toward South of Market, the streets grow more crowded with people dressed in every shade of kink, from latex to drag, grim goth to alternahip, the occasional exhibitionist wearing nothing at all. But the Folsom Street Fair began as a leather-community event, and despite the transformation of Folsom Street over the past few decades from a seedy stretch of S/M bars to a hip neighborhood filled with pricey restaurants, cowhide is still the fair's dominant fashion statement. On Folsom day, even the out-of-towners look less like they've come from Minnesota than from the ninth circle of Hell.

San Francisco, in its damned-to-hell wisdom, provides a couple of occasions suitable for heavy-duty exhibitionism. There's the Up Your Alley Fair, a pleasant afternoon among the twisted and the torturers. It is, we reassure ourselves, where the crowd remains truly hard-core, unlike the giganto Folsom fair. Harold won't be putting up his spanking booth at Folsom this year; he's so *over* the tourists pointing their digital cameras at him.

But the Folsom Street Fair is by far the larger and more notorious flesh fiesta. For many people, Folsom Sunday is the great red-letter day in the Dionysian calendar. Once upon a time, before AIDS and the invasion of the dot-coms, Folsom Street was the epicenter of the city's leather scene, a miracle mile of perversion, known around the world. These days, the former warehouse district is chockablock with trendy little clubs for the bridge-and-tunnel crowd and the live-work lofts of "artists" whose creativity expresses itself by selling pizza via the Internet. But for one glorious Sunday in September, Folsom harks back to its twisted past. The fair is the climax of "Leather Week," a time of public parties, private orgies, and, until recently, the Mr. Drummer Contest—which, following the demise of its iconic namesake, *Drummer* magazine, picked up and moved to the distinctly humid climes of South Florida; leather in Lauderdale. The studded sashes bearing the titles of semifinalists—Mr. Northwest Drummer, Southeastern Drummer Boy—are no longer in evidence, though no one seems to much mind their absence.

The fair is huge: the largest of San Francisco's many street fairs, one of the largest events of any kind in the city, packed with hundreds of thousands of folks—not just locals, but visitors from all over the country and beyond. Like Hellfire's Inferno gathering in Chicago, San Francisco's Leather Week is a Mardi Gras for the truly twisted, drawing masochists, sadists, and assorted fetishists like, inelegantly, flies to shit. It says something about San Francisco that its most popular street fair features total nudity and public floggings, but just *what* it says isn't exactly clear. To get such humongous crowds, of course, you have to appeal to more than just the hard-core kink constituency, and the Folsom Street Fair does. All sorts of people show up: leathermen and student-age twinks, pierced and tattooed hipsters and middle-class Asian-American families, the kinkerati and the most vanilla of tourists.

Unlike the Castro Street Fair, a rather chaste event held in the heart of the city's queerest neighborhood, the Folsom Street Fair just reeks of sex. The booths are less likely to be selling rainbowy *tchotchkes* than whips, paddles, and cock rings. ("Oh, look at that cute snap-on leather bracelet, dear. I want to be the first to wear one back in Des Moines.") There are public floggings, boot lickings, men mummified in duct tape or chained up against a wall. Over the years I've spotted everything from blow jobs to piss play, and I'm sure that somewhere, behind some Dumpster, a lucky guy or two has gotten fucked up the ass. It's enough to give Pat Robertson a heart attack. Or a hard-on. Who can tell with that guy?

Once past the gates of the fair, I'm swept away by a blast-furnace wave of pure, distilled lust. No matter how many times I've been there, no matter how blasé I think I am, *damn* there are some sexy men around, plenty of hidebound eye-candy on the hoof. "If I looked as good as him," I overhear one man say, "people would think I have a great personality too."

Each year, the tattoos grow more elaborate, the bodies more steroid-and-gym-bulked, the piercings more numerous and heavier-gauge. And amidst the crowd lurk the Usual Suspects: the inevitable hunky-shirtless-guy-with-a-really-big-snake-draped-around-his-shoulders; the man whose proudly displayed dick has had so much silicone injected that it looks for all the world like an illustration in a book on tropical diseases; a formidably ugly, near-naked drag queen with a flogger in each hand. Ah, yes, the Folsom Street Fair.

Perversely, grumpily, and insecurely, I usually find the non-stop flow of erotic yummies a little depressing. So this year I've wisely arranged to meet up with Nik. I figure that spending the afternoon with someone I like will be less frustrating than serious cruising would turn out to be.

Nik shows up, more or less on time, with a friend of his from high school: Pam, a big, nasty-looking, well-pierced leatherdyke. Pam tells me they went to the senior prom together, both in drag. I find myself aching to see the yearbook photos.

Pam, notwithstanding her hulking frame and her multiple piercings, turns out to be kind of shy and sweet. She's not *that* shy, however: Within a few minutes she's peeled off her shirt, revealing enormous tits with nicely pierced nipples. This being the Folsom Street Fair, breasts per se don't raise any eyebrows, but Pam's enormous mammaries draw a sidelong stare from many a leather queen. We make an odd trio, I guess: old me in chaps, skinny young Nik in his usual raggedy-boy outfit, and fireplug Pam, jugs flapping in the balmy autumn breeze.

It's early afternoon and the place is packed, block after block of self-consciously kinky hoo-ha on parade. A few of the vendors' booths offer the standard street-fair dreck, though mercifully stopping short of sand-cast candles. But most merchants are selling stuff that's still illegal in some of these freedom-loving United States: whips, dildos, paddles, piercing jewelry, restraints. It's like wandering through the workshop of some particularly evil Santa Claus. Welcome to Deviance "R" Us.

I believe—fairly devoutly—in the public display of sexuality. Not necessarily public *sex* per se. After all, even I can imagine that a family strolling through the park might not want to see butt-fucking amidst the rhododendrons; I suppose I retain enough of a shred of decency to want to spare Mom her feelings of embarrassment when Junior explains to her what's going on. But the public flaunting of private desires is an old and noble tradition, from aboriginal penis sheaths through the medieval Feast of Fools and all the way down to cute guys on MTV's *Spring Break* clad only in strategically placed shaving cream.

In olden days, a glimpse of sodomy was looked on as something shocking. But now the queer movement is underwritten by foreign automakers and distillers of overpriced vodka, cock sucking is acceptable sitcom fare, and the public face of pubic perversion is slowly but maybe inexorably changing. In the early days of post-Stonewall queerdom, the focus of the gay movement wasn't same-sex marriage or gays in the military; those assimilationist goals seemed both out of reach and beside the point. The focus back then was on what went on below the belt. I can still recall, with nostalgic fondness, marching around in some demo whilst chanting "Up the ass of the ruling class," a remarkably multileveled text that conveyed both contempt and desire, always a potent combo. The slogan unleashed our greatest threat to the homo-hating enemy: deviant desire.

I spent a small but happy fraction of my youth in bathhouse orgy pits and back-room bars' back rooms, fetid but fun places often lit by no more than one dim red bulb. They were places of indiscriminate gropings. The more ambitious among us could braille out details of clothing, hairstyle, body type. You could probably tell who had bad breath. But the only thing you could really be sure of was that the man in the adjoining darkness had a cock. This was not necessarily some paradise of love, but there were moments when the divinity of male lust was just *there*, stripped of signifiers of race, class, age, beauty. Critical mass was reached, cocks spurted, everyone zipped up and went home. Magic.

How dispiriting, therefore, to stumble across a magazine for gay and lesbian parents and discover an article in which the author bemoans the raciness of gay pride parades. We're not talking furtive blow jobs behind the beer pavilion here. The author is bent out of shape over the presence of bare-breasted Dykes on Bikes, leathermen in cowhide codpieces, drag queens.

All this is so *family-unfriendly!* We should stop it, stop it right now, before Mommy gets mad! And while we're at it, let's cut out throwing condoms to the crowd—what are little Sappho's mothers supposed to say when the dyke tyke asks what that funny balloon is for?

One might be forgiven for asking the obvious question: "What the fuck is going on here?" Here's this woman, obviously a very sincere rugmuncher, pleading that the rest of us clean up our acts for the sake of her children. "Save the children." Doesn't that sound familiar? It's one thing, dubious though it may be, to privilege what we used to call "heterocentrist values"—childbearing, monogamy, sexual restraint. It's quite another not to recognize that the very rhetoric one is using is absolutely identical to the spew of our enemies. *Have you seen their parades? What about the children, those poor innocent creatures exposed to half-naked men gyrating beside drag queens?* Religious right? Assimilationist-uptight? It makes me want to fuck someone on the roof of a lesbomom's Volvo parked at Junior's soccer game.

Fortunately, here in San Francisco our very own queer thought police haven't taken over yet. You can still say naughty words from the pride parade stage, the Radical Faeries' dicks still flop free beneath their chiffon frocks, and bare-breasted dykes still straddle their choppers (though they're *supposed* to wear Band-Aid pasties, as though their nipples were wounds). Still, even in Sodom-by-the-Bay, the contemporary queer movement is less likely to be concerned with the fate of guys busted in a freeway rest stop than in the right to inherit your partner's mutual funds.

In the midst of all this "We're just like everybody else except for what we do in bed" stuff, seeing some guy strutting down the street with his ass hanging out of his chaps still packs a salutary punch, challenging not only hetero-normative standards but the prudishness of some queers too. Which is not to say that every leather queen strutting around half dressed is on a political mission. Odds are that he's just showing off, and that's fine too.

Looking around the fair, I'm baffled—where the hell did all these perverts *come* from? From the look of things, there are enough folks into S/M to populate some small European country: Luxembourg, say. Or Liechtenstein…with whips. Of course, a number of the guys into S/M are into its "Stand & Model" variant. They're the same impossibly buff gym bunnies who'll show up a week later at the Castro Street Fair, their pumped, steroid-laden bodies squeezed into trendy shorts and overpriced T-shirts bearing the name of Calvin or Tommy or whoever this year's Abercrombie & Fitch is. But for Folsom they'll don shiny new harnesses and studded jockstraps and maybe, if you're lucky, one will stop admiring his reflection in the store windows long enough to let you give him a swat on the behind. Doubtful, but possible. Just as doubtful, actually, as his wearing that codpiece to the Castro fair, where leather, oddly, is nowhere to be seen.

Fashion versus fucking. It comes down to the difference between looking sexy and looking sexual. The first few years I went to Folsom, in my pre-kink days, I was appalled at some of what I saw there. There were old guys with saggy, dead-white bare asses hanging out of chaps. There were naked guys who were just plain fat, and assertively homely men dolled up like they were Tom of Finland models. Jesus, why didn't those guys get a clue?

Nowadays, my feelings are rather different. The men whose physiques betray hours spent at the gym when they could have been having sex seem less admirable than those less-than-perfect men who refuse to take "put that away" for an answer. "I'm here, I'm queer, I'm not stunning, and I'm horny. Get used to it," their exposed bodies seem to say. And in a society founded on sexual shame, in a "gay community" obsessed with commodified physiques, that's a message that should be yelled out loud and clear. Hip hip hooray for shamelessness, no matter how saggy its ass!

Like the spirit of carnival, the grimy dreamworld of the Folsom Street Fair grants permission. License to do what you want to do in public, even if you haven't dared to do it in private yet. And, unlike the drunk frat-boy show-us-your-tits schtick of Mardi Gras in New Orleans, Folsom is devoted to the truly down and dirty. It's a good place to try on a kinky persona and see how it feels, to strut your perversions out in the realish world. I remember one imposingly cute, bare-chested lad wearing a dog collar and leash, carrying the owner's end of the leash in his own hand. It was poignantly erection-producing, the sight of that darling li'l puppy looking for his master. I went up to talk to him—OK, to put the moves on him—and it turned out he was a total novice, had never been spanked, tied up, dominated, nothing, but there he was out there on Folsom Street, looking like your basic pigboy. False advertising, or a brave toe in the polluted lake of kink? Either way, he was uninterested in my taking him in hand. But I noticed, as the afternoon wore on and I passed him a few more times, that he was always alone, still clutching his own leash. Awww. I hope that since then, he's found someone he wants and trusts enough to give him what he seemed to be searching for. Which was, I'll venture to say, what many of us were searching for: to be overpowered, transformed, and sanctified by lust.

Yes, to stroll through the Folsom Street Fair, past the charity flogging booth and the dick-piercing-while-u-wait tent, is to become convinced that the whole wide world is into kink. This is a notion both reassuring and a bit disconcerting. It's lovely to think that just about every gay man in town is in the mood for a little abuse. And, of course, I'm all in favor of public perversion. By whomever. I think the Old Guard notion that there's an inner circle of "real" leatherfolks, surrounded by a bunch of contemptible, semi-kinky wanna-bes, is a not very edifying way to approach the world.

But there's something about the conformist coziness of the occasion that sets my contrarian teeth on edge. Part of this is no doubt due to my neuroses. When I think, *Where ARE all these pervy people the other 364 days of the year?* what I'm really thinking, I guess, is *Why won't all these attractive guys have sex with me?*

Still, not all my objections are quite so quirky. The Folsom Street Fair is an uneasy cross between an orgy and the Easter parade. Just what does perversion mean once it's tamed, put on display, and sold in little booths? Is it any more transgressive than QVC? Slings have become the macramé plant hangers of the new millennium, it seems.

On the other hand, getting the shit pleasantly beaten out of one should be one's birthright, so why be snobbishly exclusive about it? Many, maybe most queers, at least up to now, have spent their formative teenage years in a state of tumescent pariahdom. Shunned and spat on if The Secret becomes known, repressed and sulky if it remains hidden, many a gay teen finds solace in the sense that he's somehow special. "If only they knew how extraordinary I am…" the self-consolation goes. Many young queers cultivate elaborate fantasies of eventual compensatory stardom. Sprung from the cage of adolescence, plenty of mature homos still retain a teenager's desperate, uppity need to be the center of attention. Decorator queens make their homes a showplace, as though living tastefully were the best revenge. Drag queens strut around on stage in inflatable tits, vying for the title of Miss Somebody-or-Other. Muscle queens cultivate eye-popping pecs. And leather queens buy into hierarchies of butch display.

Rebellion is like that, of course. There seems to be nothing that late capitalism can't chew up and spit back out for a price. When I was a lad, responsible adults regularly pointed out that the oh-so-nonconformist hippies showed their rebellious nature by all wearing long hair and tie-dyed uniforms. These days, when trends are merchandised with the speed of light, it's even more blatant. MTV makes sure that from one corner of the globe to the other, teenage boys dress in those I-shit-in-my-pants baggy jeans or whatever the "nonconformist" trend du jour might be. The leather look was originated by the outlaw bikers of the 1950s, many of whom were indeed outlaws, often *real* outlaws whom most of us would certainly not have invited to brunch. But biker drag has become so slicked-back and overpriced that it's now the fag equivalent of all those multimillionaire Hollywood guys proving what truly butch dudes they are by putt-putting around on spotless Harleys. Jay Leno a big bad biker? Oh, puh-leeze.

It's all reminiscent of the Smothers Brothers parody of the old song "The Streets of Laredo": *I see by your outfit that you are a cowboy / I see by my outfit that I'm a cowboy too / We see by our outfits that we are both cowboys / If you get an outfit, you can be a cowboy too.* Something like that.

Faced with ample opportunities for ostentatious display, modern homos sometimes run straight the other way, into the arms of assimilation. "We're just like you hets," they smile. *Except for a desire to be fucked up the butt.* (And even that line has been crossed, the gossip goes, by increasing numbers of arrow-straight breeder guys whose rosy holes are being plowed by girlfriends with strap-ons.) Maybe the kinkiest guys in the country are running around in chinos and polo shirts, their extreme sexual tastes invisible to the naked eye. I, with my love of the unexpected, kind of hope so.

One of the ways I survived high school was by being brainier than almost everybody else. I was busy reading William Burroughs and Susan Sontag long before I should have even heard of *The New York Review of Books*. This perhaps explains why, descending into the bacchanal of the Folsom Street Fair, I spend entirely too much time pondering the meaning of it all instead of trying to get laid.

If I were breathtakingly handsome or blindingly drunk, I'd be braver at these events. Even so, I've had my fun at the fairs. There was that tall, kind of geeky man with a big nose, wearing nothing but Converse sneakers and a jockstrap, who made out with me outside a leather bar. I pinned him up against a street sign and we sucked face whilst I spanked his naked ass till it grew warm and gratifyingly pink. (This is, let me hasten to point out to the fastidious among you who've never been to such events, not at all viewed as misbehavior.) By the time we made it into the bar my hand was in his jockstrap, and once inside the bar his jock slipped to his ankles, revealing shaved pubes and a gratifyingly pretty cock. (And I suppose somewhere along the line he gave me head, though the ol' memory's not what it used to be.) Every year since, I've seen him near-naked at Folsom, though he doesn't recognize me. Ah well. So much for love.

Then there was the Romanian Dentist. I didn't know he was a Romanian, or even a dentist, when we met. The fair was drawing to a close when I spotted him, blandly handsome, somehow Slavic, watching a spanking demonstration. He looked as vanilla as they get, but something about him read "corruptible."

"Looks like fun, huh?" I opened, inanely.

"Yes, it does," he replied, in heavily accented high school English.

He was a dentist from Bucharest, visiting his sister in Silicon Valley. And yes, he repeated, the spanking looked like fun. But seeing as how I couldn't invite him back to my place, and he had no place to go, would I care to walk him back to his car?

Within 20 minutes we were in a Honda Civic—his sister's car, actually—parked right outside the Eagle, San Francisco's venerable leather bar. (Venerable leather bars *anywhere* are, more often than not, called the Eagle.) And I was pounding away on his cock and balls. The Romanian Dentist, mild-mannered and dweeby, had turned out to be into cock-and-ball torture big time. The guy, your basic ordinary-looking who'd-have-thunk-it fella, was a pain pig par excellence. To one side of the Honda, leathermen were promenading from the fair to the bar. On the other side, SUVs full of suburbanites were whizzing by, heading toward the freeway. And there we were—me slapping, him squirming in pleasure. I loved the possibility that the scene we were doing could be observed not only by burly guys in chaps, but by Johnny and Grandma headed back to Palo Alto after a day at Fisherman's Wharf. Since the Romanian Dentist kept his pants on, I doubt we'd even violated any laws, except, that is, the Stern and Eternal Law of God—who indulges His own sadistic impulses by, say, destroying the Cities of the Plain. And what made it all special, what catapulted the scene from "fun" to "transcendent," was the bloody unlikelihood of it all. The fair, the wild feast of leather fools, had moved past the barricades into what's laughingly called "the real world."

Did some of the leathermen swaggering by see what was going on in the car with the fogged-up windows? How could they not? Did some right-winger in a Chevy glance over to see me whacking on the dentist's crotch? Shit, I sure hope so.

Some weeks later, I discovered that the bottom from Bucharest had cut quite a kinky swath during his sojourn, spending a big chunk of his Bay Area vacation whoring around with assorted sadists. When I told the story at a dinner party, it turned out that three friends of mine had worked him over too. Within certain circles, one had only to utter the words "Romanian dentist" for the reference to be clear.

This year, though, even without the dentist, the presence of Nik and Pam is providing plenty of diversion. Nik is living proof that I'm sexually attractive to at least one guy I find irresistible, while Pam's big lesbian tits draw the attention of gay boys and dykes alike. And somewhere along the line, after a beer or two and a bit of weed, I drop the analysis, the competitiveness, the insecure envy of the gorgeous, the coveting of $300 whips, and I just have *fun*—a good dirty old time. Which is, damn it, what it's all supposed to be about. When we stop at the Lesbian Avengers' "Have Your Photo Taken with a Dyke for a Buck" booth, one willowy gay boy insists on having his photo taken with Pam, his hand hoisting one of her mammoth mammaries, a big grin on his face. The Lesbian Avengers get the dollar.

The Folsom Street Fair winds down, as always, into a late-afternoon swirl of discarded beer cups, last-minute discounts on sex toys, and wasted men pissing in Porta Pottis or, more rarely but pleasingly, on each other. By the next morning it will be hard to say just what has been gained, except for a holiday from repressive sanity, and in some cases, perhaps, a persistent case of crabs. But for the time being, as Nik and I hug and say goodbye and Pam tugs her T-shirt over her commodious breasts, everything seems ragged but right. We have joined—all of us, the whipmasters and the wanna-bes, the merely crazed and the truly insane—in a celebration of Eros triumphant, the kind of bacchanal that would make respectable gay and lesbian parents wince. Those of them, that is, who haven't left the kids with a sitter, slipped on chaps and a harness, and headed on down to the Folsom Street Fair.

CHAPTER 11
Macho, Macho Man:
Leather Contests and Other Butch Pursuits

If you hang around S/M-ers long enough, the lustful quest for twisted pleasure can start to look like a rather odd little contest. Who can take the most pain? Who's top dog with a single-tailed whip? Whose bondage skills are best, and who's a mere perv poseur? This competitive cocksmanship takes its most obvious, most banal form in the world of leather competitions. Whether his title is International Mr. Leather, Mr. Drummer, or some other Mr. Something, the sash-wearing winner of a leather contest is part ravening sadomasochist, part pert Miss America.

In 1997 I was assigned to cover the Mr. Drummer Contest, writing an article for its namesake and then-sponsor, the now-defunct grandaddy of the leather magazines, *Drummer*. The annual shindig was, back then, a big fucking San Franciscan deal, at least among those of us who like our studs to wear studs.

At the pre-contest Basket Auction, the back room of the Powerhouse Bar is hectic with regional Mr. Drummers arranging their fund-raising displays of goods to be auctioned off, displays of dildos, lube, and porn videos arranged just so. It's like a bunch of students preparing their homeroom for Parents' Night, except that these students have great chests, bulging crotches, and mostly black outfits in which various lengths of chain figure prominently.

I strike up a conversation with Mr. Florida Drummer, whose naked ass is (not coincidentally) one of the most perfect butts of all time. He's charming, with a ready smile that I can only describe (sorry, machismo worshipers) as adorable. As he tells me of his years of preparation leading up to this week, my eyes keep drifting down to his leather-and-chrome–clad crotch. I'm glad not to be one of the contest judges, who'll have to maintain Olympian impartiality: I already know whom I'll be rooting for.

A few days later contest time rolls around. When I walk in from a sunny mid-afternoon, Club Townsend seems as dark as Jesse Helms's soul. The VIP crowd, coed, multiracial, and multigenerational, from Old Guard guys with wrinkles to a kid with a magenta Mohawk, is chowing down on free food and beer. It has the conviviality of a Sunday afternoon at the Eagle bar but with a minimum of cruising and a maximum of networking. Which is not to say that there aren't some incredibly hot guys here. But there's no back room and little groping. There isn't even a trace of tit torture.

I run into Mr. Florida Drummer again. He's still friendly, still cute, and assures me he wouldn't mind being described as "adorable." Dang, I'm in love.

Eventually the hoi polloi file in and the perverted proceedings get under way. A cross between the Shriners and an orgy, the world of the leather contest strikes a tone of self-congratulation which, given leatherfolks' record of charitable endeavors, is well-deserved. Still, amidst all that high-minded talk, it's sometimes easy to lose sight of the fact that this is really all about a bunch of guys who like to put clothespins on other men's dicks. And vice versa.

For those of you not fortunate enough to have witnessed a leather title competition, be assured that it runs to the familiar model of your basic beauty pageant. There are the "if I'm elected, here's how I'll save the world" speeches; the talent competition, though more likely to focus on flogging than baton twirling; and then there's the swimsuit, er, jockstrap parade.

After an initial intro to the aspirants, it's time to get acquainted with the hunks in harnesses. The candidates' speeches are fairly pro forma. Let's face it: Nobody's going to get up and say, "I don't give a fuck about humanity. I just like slapping around other guys till they squirm." There are proprieties to be observed. I start to squirm. With impatience.

The baton twirling comes next—this particular talent contest features the boys acting out little S/M skits. The fantasies are pretty interesting, though they tend to bring out my inner drama critic; most of the acting vacillates between porn video and high school play. One surprise: A couple of the contestants present themselves as heavy bottoms, one of them being fake-fisted by an ancient Egyptian priest, the other getting screwed by Santa Claus. And Mr. Northern California Drummer's comic skit of running a misfiring scene fraught with broken paddles, falling-apart floggers, and a collapsing St. Andrew's cross brings a huge response from the tops in the audience, folks who know what performance anxiety is all about.

I'm not surprised at the lack of genital nudity onstage, since booze is being served—liquor laws, y'know. But whatever S/M schtick there is tends to be Kink Lite: a couple of slaps here, a bit of bondage there. A nice hot-wax scene leaves the sadist in me panting for more, but then intermission rolls around.

Time to cruise. Considering they're at an event for which sex is the raison d'être, it's a remarkably restrained bunch. But friendly, with an undercurrent of "look you over now, fuck you later." And there's plenty to look at. A tall young guy with a way-spankable ass sticking out of his chaps. A hairy Daddy with a great dick taking a piss at the next urinal. Lots more.

The folks at the magazine have told me they want me to come up with something sleazy for my article. Even so, I never do check out the rumor about the water-sports bottom in the end stall of the ladies' room, assuming that my informant was pulling my leather-clad leg. If you want to imagine, though, that intermission at the Mr. Drummer Contest featured a guy sprawled belly-up on a toilet, legs in the air, while a steady succession of leathermen emptied recycled beer down his thirsty throat, gushing till it cascaded over his torso and soaked his pulsating asshole, then by all means, dear reader, be my guest.

OK, back to the show. Part Two features not one but two fantasies in which fisters pull funny things out of a bottom's butt. And two fantasies featuring the ever-butch Mickey Mouse. Some trends are definitely shaping up. If only I were able to figure out what the fuck they mean.

The big hit, though, is my pal Mr. Florida's fantasy. He plays Peter Pansexual, flying with a transgendered Wendy to Leather-Leather Land. The crowd eats it up. I begin to think that being adorable might have its rewards after all.

The jock strap competition goes by in a flash. We've already seen quite a lot of the guys' bodies anyhow, so perhaps a more titillating wet-Jockey-shorts contest would have been more of a giggle than this cowhide-and-studs parade. I do find it reassuring that the contestants aren't all Falcon Video–perfect but instead reflect the way that leatherfolk value a variety of body types, from buff to bearish.

One final fantasy (one where a rainbow flag gets pulled out of a bottom's butt, Mickey Mouse being mercifully absent), and then it's vote-counting time.

Another sleaze-free intermission. I toy with the idea of dashing to the back-room bar up the street to get my cock sucked but opt for journalistic integrity instead. I ask myself the hard questions. *How can a room full of half-naked homos*, I ponder, *remain so damn well-behaved?*

At last the big moment is on its way. In his farewell speech the previous year's winner seems intent on settling some old scores; amidst all the blather about "community," the bitchery actually seems endearingly honest.

And then the climax of any awards show, the opening of the envelopes. A crowd favorite, Northern California Drummerboy, clinches the Drummerboy title. The Golden Whip Award, awarded by the contestants themselves to the guy who best upholds the Leather Tradition, is awarded to Mr. Florida Drummer. (Think of it as Miss Congeniality with a cock.) *So I'm not the only one who likes him,* I think. *Maybe he'll get the Big One.* The suspense is, well, palpable. Second runner-up, Troy Taylor. First runner-up, John Brown. And International Mr. Drummer 1997 is…Mr. Florida Drummer, Jeffrey Adler.

Much to my surprise, I find myself leaping to my feet and yelling "YEAH!" Thank God I don't pump my fist in the air. After the inevitable photo op, I go onstage to congratulate the winner. And to thank him for providing such a good ending to my article. And I kiss him. Sure, I've kissed many a man before, but never a titleholder. Gosh.

So that's that for another year, the crowd drifting into the warm early evening. And I find myself, maybe surprisingly, believing that the International Mr. Drummer competition was pretty much what it set out to be. A celebration of the intersection of flesh and fantasy. A reinvigoration of the soul of a community that, despite some pretty rough times, has persevered and thrived. And a welcome confirmation that I know a nice piece of ass when I see it.

Once upon a time, way back in the mid-20th century, homosexuality was generally viewed as a gender disorder: Faggots were men who wanted to be women. The sissy archetype was all that most straights understood. There was, even then, a hypermasculine underground of leathermen, but it was a genuinely sub-rosa subculture, what's now dubbed "Old Guard." After Stonewall, though, more and more gay men realized that they could be just as masculine (or more so) as the straight down the street. Rather than gay men being seen as sissies seeking real men to provide the masculinity they themselves lacked, the guy-guy coupling could be viewed as all-male terrain, a place where masculine desires came out to play, untainted by the female of the species. Tom of Finland, the porn painter who celebrated near-fascist masculine icons, all bulging muscles and even more oversize cocks, went from underground notoriety to mainstream stardom in coffee-table art books. Yet even Tom's butch boys betrayed voluptuous disjunctures; their chisel-jawed faces were *too* perfect, too pretty, their eyes hinting at mascara, their immaculately tousled hair gleaming with Brylcreem. Their "unforced" masculinity was, pretty clearly, performative. They were male impersonators.

I'm far from the first person to point out that gay men who butch it up in defiance of sissifying stereotypes are, ironically, measuring themselves by the very same standards of gender that oppress them. (Flaming queens do the same sort of thing too, though in a backflip: "You say that I'm a fag? *I'll* show you how big a fag I can *be*, you asshole!")

There are men who are into leather and not S/M, and vice versa, but the combo of kink and cowhide is a potent one. There's a tribal bonding that's cemented by endurance-based rites of passage, just like in New Guinea…kind of. Somewhere along the line, spurred by big-time pervs like Fakir Musafar, the godfather of the piercing craze, the parallels became explicit. The late Geoff Mains wrote an influential book, *Urban Aboriginals*, that cast leathermen as members of a tribe. The phrase *Modern*

Primitives gained currency, and suddenly everyone and his queer uncle was getting tattooed and pierced in the most unlikely places. Every small town, it seemed, had a tattoo and piercing place, just down the street from Applebee's.

Sure, Modern Primitives and the rest of the pervert bunch include women, het men, and various other genders, not just homo men. But the position of the gay leatherman is particularly fraught. One of the homophobes' Big Accusations is that gay men are self-indulgent pleasure sluts. Now, to some of *us*, that doesn't sound like a major sin. But *manly* men, the story goes, sublimate their lust. In the Western World at least, stoic self-denial is a major signifier of masculinity. Real (read "straight") men manage to keep their pussy lust in check, at least in theory. Giving in to emotions and desires is something *women* do, fer chrissakes. Homophobic discourse around sexuality doesn't equate heterosexuality with fucking but with "family," the conversion of anarchic lust into a stable unit of production. Sexual self-denial: It's the manly thing to do.

Not all gay men are sluts, of course. Some of us are celibate, some monogamous, and as long as these choices are made out of genuine desire, not insecurity or fear, they're just fine. But a significant proportion of us are not only hot to trot, but we trot a lot more frequently than the usual rules of male-female courtship allow most straight men to do. Hell, we're already outcasts, so if we want, we get to break a *lot* of rules. And S/M desires, in particular, find fulfillment in all sorts of cool and unusual punishments.

S/M is about pleasure of course, but it's also about vulnerability and mastery—not just mastery of another person but above all mastery of oneself. Gay leathermen prove their masculinity by taking punishment with a stiff upper lip or dishing it out with a sneer. But unlike football or war, with their submerged homobonding, gay S/M shoves the sexuality up front for everyone to see. And unlike het male bullying, the power games are tender collaborations. When leathermen play, they're focused laserlike on queer desire and ruled by the whip hand of lust, which makes them, in the eyes of the anti-gay, less than really real men, no matter how much they strut or suffer.

Newcomers to leather culture often go to their first play party expecting randy, overmuscled studs fucking one another with appropriately immense cocks. What a surprise, then, to find that a whole lot of leathersex has little or nothing to do with dick. S/M players not only might not cum, they might not even be hard. The site of desire is diffused over the whole body: Cocks are made to be tortured, true, but so are tender nipples, bulging buttocks, shoulders, pecs. If maleness is supposedly phallic, then how to approach a form of sexuality that, though embracing the hypermasculine, often downplays the dick? (Yes, this is the kind of abstruse question that fascinates queer theorists, who make whole careers out of obscure academic noodlings about cock. But bear with me for a sec.)

The leather-clad body of the top is *all* dick, erect and armored, ready for hard action. The bottom is all hole, ready to receive the top's thrusting power. In a lot of gay S/M play, the dick is everywhere but nowhere. For all the butch rituals, the leathermale just ain't so phallocentric. The ultramale endurance rituals are also, paradoxically, displays of radical vulnerability, the kind of thing that might be called "feminine." (Bottoms? Pussyboys.) And so gay leathersex both celebrates and challenges stereotypical masculinity. Or something like that.

I once saw a great sign in the gay pride parade: IT TAKES A REAL MAN TO WEAR A DRESS. Well, mebbe, mebbe not. But gay S/M, though all dressed up in chaps, challenges (in weirdly subversive and usually unacknowledged ways) standard gender roles.

Notwithstanding the supermacho conventions of leather porn and the rampant misogyny of some gay leathermen, the paradoxes of the leather scene are a dead-on deconstruction of traditional masculinity. The theatricalization of "butch," no matter how seriously it's taken by leathermen, provides a case study in gender-as-performance. Traditional maleness becomes just another fetish, and if beneath that storm trooper's uniform there lurks a hairdresser who adores Puccini, well, that's showbiz. Sure, there are some "naturally" hypermasculine guys who don't change their tone when they put on black leather, but even that supposedly unfeigned butchness has to come from somewhere, right? "Cigar smoker" is not a genetic trait.

Both inside and out of the leather community, there's often a denigration of effeminacy that can not only be oppressive but raises suspicions. If, as the truism has it, homophobia stems from a fear of being queer oneself, then where does sissyphobia come from, huh?

Still, many leathermen are actually pretty secure about the ironies of gay machismo. One of the more telling rituals of leather culture is an event that's called "The Leather and Lace Contest" or something similar. At the heart of the competition, big butch leathermen transform themselves into gorgeous drag queens, and a good time is had by all. And, in San Francisco at least, leather events are more likely to be adorned by the male nuns of the Sisters of Perpetual Indulgence or drag queens with too-clever names than by "straight-acting" boys in chinos.

Which is not to say that the actual "leather community," for all its charitable good works, is a particularly progressive force. It's often said that leathermen are significantly more right-wing than the queer community at large, and I've seen some argue that female-to-male transsexuals should be barred from their play parties, as though they were at a mirror image of the

Michigan Womyn's Music Fest. But I've found that the most experienced leathermen are less likely to guard their oh-so-butch image than those on the fringes of the scene, so perhaps S/M play does grant androgynous insights. After all, what matters most is pain, pleasure, and power, not prick or pussy.

It's not merely the religious right that gets the willies when a man with a whip strolls by. Assorted assimilationists and Respectable Gay Leaders have decried the presence of leather-men in pride parades. They've come down on drag queens too, but that makes a certain (though bigoted) sense, since guys in fishnets might be seen as reinforcing the stereotype of fags as would-be women. But if we're *not* all sissies, then why not spot-light the butchest-looking of us all? Why not encourage Tom of Oakland to light up that stogie, pull on his chaps, and clomp down Main Street in his big black boots? Why not show to all the world that real men take it up the ass?

What's everybody afraid of?

CHAPTER 12
That's SIR to You: Masters and Slaves

I'm seeing a very cute sub boy who has aspirations to slavery. He's a clerk at a chain bookstore, and I suppose that's a start. Previously I'd shied away from anything that even suggested contractual slavery, but I am, it should be clear by now, pretty much helpless where desire is concerned. And this boy, the Clerk, looks utterly adorable in a leather collar. He seems eager to play too; every time he comes over and strips down, his adorable little cock is already hard and dripping-wet. So I figure I might do him a favor and draw up a part-time slavery contract. Since he has a boyfriend and is sneaking around behind his partner's back, I'm assuming there's an extremely limited future to his "slavery," but there *is* that cute hard-on...

The Clerk also has a pal who works at the same store. Clerk 2, it seems, is fascinated by Clerk's tales of what he and I have done. Clerk 2 fancies himself a Total Top, Clerk told me, but has yet to actually do anything that isn't pure vanilla. Would it be OK, they both wonder, if Clerk 2 were to serve as my apprentice, the two of us dominating my "slave"?

Well, yeah, maybe, but I want to get to know Clerk 2 first. So Clerk gives him my phone number, and a call follows shortly thereafter. Clerk 2, it turns out, has gotten a lot of his notions about kink from reading Camille Paglia, always a bad sign as far as I'm concerned. He has, it turns out, pretty elaborate ideas about who he is and what he's after. Clerk 2 has decided he's a dominant, sadistic personality who wants—no, *deserves*—a full-time slave, someone who'll attend to his every erotic need, serve him, and give him pleasure. I figure it sounds like he's just looking for a good, attentive top, but I am not about to disabuse him of his notion of Mastery.

We arrange to meet at his place, then go for a walk or grab some coffee, just to feel one another out. When I get to his flat, Clerk 2 turns out to look a bit like my first boyfriend, if my first boyfriend had been blond and had suffered from a medium-bad case of adult acne. He is, in fact, damn good-looking, and I can't decide whether the acne adds to his attractiveness by making him seem less perfect. He's wearing what my long-ago boyfriend would have worn: a black turtleneck, fairly tight jeans, boring shoes. Clerk 2 looks less like an S/M Master than a librarian. Or a bookstore clerk.

I like him.

I also want him, and I figure if he's too uptight to let me touch him, the proposed three-way won't work out at all. So, tentatively, I touch him. I have to confess that part of me is hoping he'll lash out like the tightly wound beast he believes himself to be, throw me to the carpet, and grind his boring black shoe into my submissive crotch.

Not a chance. Of course.

Clerk Number 2, to my almost total lack of surprise, turns out to be a great big bottom. Of course. It's not that I'm a fabulously dominant man; I'm not, but I've been around the sexual-needs block more than a few times, and I can figure out some things pretty quick. Within moments I have him pinned to the bed by his wrists, holding down his straining, humping body, hard-on and all.

I have, actually, a great time. Not the best topping I've ever done, but certainly fun. I try several times to reach under his turtleneck or to pull it off entirely. No dice; I guess his acne is pretty bad. When I tug at his shirt he looks like he's going to cry. Poor, scared Masterboy. But soon enough, naked from the waist down, having been shoved around and spanked a bit, Clerk 2 shoots his wad. I suspected the afterwards might be emotionally messy, and it is. I've sussed him out. He's been busted. I know where he's coming from: He has such issues with his body that he wouldn't take his damn shirt off, not even when he was having sex. He's figured, I guess, that no one who wasn't an utter sub slave would ever actually put out for him, to give him the attention and affirmation he clearly, oh so clearly, craves. And here I've made him, maybe for the first time in his life, the absolute center of a sex scene. I have a feeling of triumph, and it's tinged with self-congratulation, not contempt. I find myself thinking, "Tell *that* to Camille Fucking Paglia."

Needless to say, after that Clerk 2 and I never do end up co-topping Clerk 1. Oh well, I'd obligingly done my best to make my "slave"-to-be's dreams come true. I'm *such* a nice sadist.

I do draw up a slavery contract for Clerk 1, one that only applies to his behavior when we're actually in contact, either on the phone or playing in person. I put in all the things I figure should go into such a formal document: stuff about his addressing me as "Sir," his keeping his eyes downcast, his immediately disrobing in my presence unless instructed to do otherwise. You know, all that good porno stuff. I figure it won't have the force of law. At least I hope not. Who wants to be taken to small-claims court over cock sucking?

Once I have the contract written up and thoroughly copy-edited, I print it out in a suitably Gothic face and invite, er, command Clerk to come over to my place for the signing ritual. Stripped-down, collared, with that cute little hard-on that just won't quit leaking, Clerk kneels before Masterful me as I go over each of the contractual clauses, one by one. Instead of merely respectfully nodding at each provision, though, he takes advantage of my offer to discuss things, fretting about each detail as though his freedom depends on it. I suppose you could have made a case for his integrity—would-be Slave Clerk wanting to be sure he understood and could live up to his commitment before signing himself over into part-time servitude. Then as now, though, the whole thing just smacked of ingratitude. Last time I looked, *submissive* didn't mean "arranged exactly the way I like it." I'd thought I was going to take possession of a bookstore clerk, but I end up wrangling with a contract lawyer instead. Pushy bottoms are bad enough. But pushy *slaves*? Oh, give me a break. Please.

Anyway, after a long, long, long discussion, we sign the thing, and go on to play for a while, during which the details of the contract seem not to matter at all. Ah, well, give the slaveboy time to do his homework.

"So," I say, as we're pulling on our clothes, "here's your copy of the contract to take home and study."

"Listen," says my property, "I'm afraid if I take it with me, my boyfriend will find it. Can't you just keep my copy too, and I'll look at it again next time I'm here?"

I suppose I let out an audible sigh. If not, I should have.

And that is, to my not-entirely-great surprise, the last time I ever see my slave naked. He's never given me his phone number— the boyfriend thing, you know. My E-mails go unanswered. A Slavemaster has his pride, you know, or at least I guess He's supposed to, but after several weeks of nonresponsive silence from my utterly obedient contractual part-time slave, I stop by the bookstore where he works. And there at the register is Clerk 2, the would-be Master.

"Hi," I say, "where's Clerk?"

"He's working over at that desk," said the handsome-but-acned Paglia fan, looking somewhat disconcerted. I wonder whether he feels the slightest bit of regret for never having returned my phone calls after his big adventure in bottoming. Or if he regrets ever meeting me in the first place. Often in a post-tricking situation those two regrets are hard to tell apart.

I walk across the store. Sure enough, Clerk is there, as impossibly cute as ever.

"I've been meaning to call you," he says, "but my boyfriend situation has been sort of weird."

I might, if I want to be legalistic about it, remind him that he has a contractual obligation to at least reply to my fucking E-mail. Instead, I say, "OK, get in touch when you have some clear time."

And that—no surprise—is pretty much it. I'm not about to go mooning over two pieces of meat whose submissiveness runs neck and neck with their boyish ingratitude. Well, all right, I do moon over them, but tastefully restrain myself from ever strolling into Borders, throwing myself on the floor, and whining to the Clerks, "Please, please, be my slaves again. Oh ple-e-e-ase…"

That sort of thing is just not done. Not even by me.

A couple of months later my parents are in town, staying near the bookstore, and I drag them in there to see a couple of new anthologies my work is in. And there's little Clerk, looking thoroughly adorable. My heart gives a little leap composed equally of joy and irritation. It does seem nicely transgressive to introduce my parents to a boy who'd promised to be my sex slave. But then I start to think of the whole Master/slave schtick's parallels to conventional marriage, and it makes me want to giggle. Or to drag Clerk over my knee and spank his silly ass.

That's the last time I see him. He never, ever gets in touch again. Every once in a while I stop into Borders to see if the boys are around, but eventually I give up; from what I hear, personnel turnover there is pretty high. But then, as I found out firsthand, it's so hard to retain good servants nowadays.

Porn classics like John Preston's *Mr. Benson* or Laura Antoniou's *Marketplace* trilogy have launched countless wet-dream fantasies of utter subservience. The slave, a homebound sex object supported and dominated by a rich, butch man, keeps house all day, and is there kneeling, naked and collared, when Master comes home. To some folks, this and only this is the true goal toward which all dominance scenes point; anything less is makeshift. To me, there's a thin line between "perfect slave" and "perfect wife," but maybe that's just sour grapes. Clearly, the idea of surrendering one's will to a more powerful person who'll care for you, discipline you, and free you from the burdens of freedom has powerful attractions. It may not even be an aping of traditional het male-on-top marriage. It might go deeper than that: a desire to return to childhood. Daddy will keep you fed and sheltered, and all you have to do is finish your chores and not misbehave.

That's the appeal for the bottom, of course. Likewise, to the putative Master, the idea of total ownership, body and soul, of another human being does have a certain tasty tang. Holy cow, who wouldn't want to be King of the Castle? And so the fantasy has a real durability. For a while I was fascinated by the possibility that the phenomenon of a consensual, contractual Master/slave relationship, full-fledged, full-time, was the real thing and not, like crop circles, merely a clever hoax dreamed up to hornswoggle the rubes.

There's the little matter of class, of course—few of my friends can even pay off their credit card bills, never mind owning a slave. But maybe, in the stratospheric reaches of the A-gay super-rich, some Hollywood mogul or trust-fund zillionaire actually hangs out in some Marketplace buying up a hunk or two at MasochistMart. What do I know?

Oh, I'm sure they're out there somewhere: real honest-to-God slaves, 24/7 submissives just like in the porn stories. Thoroughly selfless pieces of meat whose one and only desire is to serve their masters well. If you're one of them, don't take offense. Please. Like I said, I'm sure you're out there somewhere. I just haven't met any of you, is all.

My next run-in with a would-be slave started innocuously enough. I was at a play party at the usual dungeon. My friend Barton had a guy tied to the rack. Bottom's body looked great. His face, covered with a gas mask, was an unknown. Barton is a nice enough fellow with a really nice cock, but he isn't what you'd call a bondage maven. So when I came along and evinced interest, he willingly handed the scene over to me.

I go to work, wrapping more rope around the stranger's body, cinching it tight, tighter. The only part I can see of my bottom's face is his eyes, glinting with pleasure through the mask. That's quite enough.

We play till the party winds down, then we play a little longer. It is, as are many pure bondage scenes, something of a Taoist affair. You can do all sorts of colorful, nasty things to tied-up guys, of course, but the essence of bondage is immobility, a dark calm in the middle of all those ropes and geegaws. At last I pull off the gas mask to reveal a handsome man in his 30s, an Englishman named Daniel. "I'm all yours, Sir," he says.

Some guys are into bondage as foreplay. But pure bondage bottoms long to be tied down not so they can be "forced" into that which they fervently desire, but because, well, they want to be tied down. And this guy appears to be as pure a bondage bottom as I've ever buckled my collar on.

I know the guys who own the dungeon, and with their permission Daniel and I spend the night there. He, hands and feet bound, sleeps in my arms, and when we awake we play some more. After a few hours we take a break and swap autobiographies. Daniel tells me this is his next-to-last day in San Francisco for a while. He's flying back to Britain, but he'll back in the fall, first spending several months doing motivational training for the employees of a famous Silicon Valley firm, then doing some traveling around the States.

Just my fucking luck. I find the perfect bottom, and he's got a plane ticket out.

When I go home for lunch I pack my video camera, and once back at Daniel's hotel room I gleefully shoot him "struggling" against his ropes, uncut dick swollen purple, his writhing punctuated by frequent moans. We spend most of his remaining time together, playing long into the night. This is, clearly, as good as it gets. Amazing. When I see him off on the airport van the next morning, we exchange pledges to wait for one other until autumn rolls around.

It doesn't take long before I begin getting letters from him, postmarked London. "I got tied up last weekend," one of them says, "but at the other end of the ropes, all I saw was you." Each of us wants to be special. Having someone love us is one way. Being sexually desired is another. S/M tops want to hear that they're The Best, the most skilled, most dominant. They want someone who'll believe that. And bingo, I'd found him, my Slave of a Lifetime, my number one fan.

I write back, trying to be both enthusiastic and realistic. But Daniel's letters start getting a little…overwhelming.

"I want you to know that there are no limits between us, that my trust in you is absolute, my surrender complete."

On the basis of one long fuck session? Whoa! I don't know

who he thinks he's talking to, but whoever it is, it sure ain't me.

Still, he's undeniably hot-looking and was a total pleasure to play with. Every so often I throw the tape I've shot into the VCR and watch Daniel in bondage. God, that uncut cock, all tied up…what a masturbatory dream! But when I panned up to his face, I now notice, Daniel exhibited an easily readable self-consciousness. He was, visibly, less a submissive lost in the throes of ecstasy than someone *pretending* to be "a submissive lost in the etc."

In late August, just weeks before the long-anticipated Return of the Slave, I get a call from my friend Bob, whom I've told all about Daniel. "That English boy of yours?" Bob asks. "What's his name again?"

I tell him.

"Thought so," Bob says. "I've been reading his posts on this Internet newsgroup I subscribe to. He's been advertising for a full-time Master. And it looks like he's found one."

I've been diddled. Cuckolded by the man whose devotion to me was, he'd sworn, absolute. So much for "total submission." And Daniel is due back in San Francisco soon.

Just days before his arrival, I get another letter. "This is so hard to say," runs the familiar handwriting, "but I have to tell you I've found a Master, a strong, wonderful man who lives in Los Angeles. I've signed a year-long slavery contract with him, and I'll only be able to see you with his permission. I'm so very sorry." Yeah, I'll just bet.

As attracted to Daniel as I might have been before, now that he's out of reach I'm totally obsessed. My feelings are a mess. I hate him because he's betrayed me. I hate myself because I'm not enough of a top to hold him, not enough of a real man. I hate his Master, I hate the game, I hate my willingness to be taken for a big old roller-coaster ride. And I hate knowing that, if Daniel were to call and tell me it's all been a mistake, I would forgive him in an instant. Come back to me, slaveboy. Stupid, stupid, stupid.

But then, desire is stupid.

I see Daniel once shortly after his return, hurriedly, in his new white Toyota, meeting me in defiance of his new Master's rules, a Master he's yet to meet face-to-face. Daniel is still, yes, so beautiful, so desirable. And my disappointment, my disaster. "It's just that your letters to me had seemed so…hesitant. So I looked elsewhere."

But you promised! I want to say. I don't, though. Real tops don't whine.

In the days that follow, things go from bad to worse. Daniel flies to L.A. for the weekend. I call him that Monday to see how things have gone with his new Master.

"I told my Sir what I'd done, meeting you without his permission. He beat me like I'd never been beaten before. It was wonderful."

My throat tightens in a confusion of envy, desire, and utter incomprehension of how things could have gone so wrong. One minute I'd been masterful Master of all Daniel's dreams, the next a pitiful also-ran.

He re-explains it for me, though. "I apologize for all this. It's just that your letters…they weren't what I needed to hear."

And there you have it. I hadn't followed the script.

If I were wise, I'd walk away and not look back. Away from the manipulations, untruths, self-deceptive falsehoods. But I'm a slave to the lure of unfufillable desire. If unrequited lust is the drug, I'm well and truly hooked. What a squalid mess. My partner hears me kvetch about Daniel so often he's tempted to throw me out. And the soap opera gets still worse. Stupider. Daniel's L.A. top, MASTER Jeff (in Daniel's letters, the title always got all caps) keeps changing the rules.

Daniel can't meet with me at all. Then he can't phone me, I have to phone him. Then he's not permitted to return my phone messages. I'm Passion's Plaything, pathetically caught up in a leather-bound edition of *Les Liaisons Dangereuses*. At one point I even write MASTER Jeff a letter, explaining that I'm not, I swear, a threat to his MASTERful hegemony, and could I please, please see Daniel? Please? And thus doth passion make pussies of us all.

The letter I get back from MASTER Jeff fairly drips with scorn. It's greasy with contempt. Lucky for Daniel, says Jeff, that he escaped getting involved with a not-very-masterful loser like me.

I'm all at sea, utterly befuddled by own incompetence, my evident lack of topitude. I *want* to believe in the mythos. I want there to be a world of deep, dark devotion. But all I can see is low-level game-playing, the kind that schoolyard bullies and their adoring minions engage in. Or maybe—could it be?—I'm just being defensive, covering for my overwhelming failures as a sadist, a top, an S/M player and, clearly, a Man. Or at least a Manly Man who deserves a boy on a leash. The absolute bathetic nadir comes when I go to see *Madame Butterfly* at the opera. I sit there crying copiously, mourning not the fate of delicate Cio-cio-San but the tragic end of Daniel and Simon's kinky affair. Jesus!

In my quest to make sense of things, I've started reading a lot of S/M porn, though that, it soon becomes clear, is a mistake; most of that over-the-top smut stuff is no closer to recognizable real life than *Star Trek*. I begin to ask around, but none of my kinky friends actually knows a couple in a strict, contractual, live-in 24/7 Master/slave relationship. But then most of my friends have a tough enough time making ends meet, never mind having the disposable shekels to keep a slaveboy in gruel and harnesses. If there *is* a Mr. Benson, he no doubt lives in Bel Air.

Finally, I figure I'll ask the person who, if anyone could explain things, would be the one: Pat Califia, the acknowledged master of power-based porn. I phone up Pat, who's not only a wonderful writer and a fine person but a professional counselor too. I explain the situation. "Pat, I just don't know what to think about all this…"

And Pat, with the bullshit-cutting clarity of a Zen monk thwacking a disciple on the noggin, says, "Simon, I would never have a full-time slave. *It's just too much work.*"

And I am immediately enlightened. The scales drop from my eyes with a crash. Daniel, I finally realize (albeit with the slightly vicious edge of the jilted lover), does not want to be a slave, surrendering his body and will to another. He wants to *pretend* to be a slave. What he really wants to be is a kid, one whose Daddy will play cowboys and Indians with him whenever sonny boy wants, and who will always let him win. Not that there's nothing *wrong* with playing Let's Pretend, as long as you're aware you're doing it. Otherwise, it's schizophrenia.

I never see my runaway slaveboy after that. And I hardly even care. I might have lost, but I did get a handful of lovely consolation prizes.

First off, the whole fucked-up situation has taught me a lot, and hard-won wisdom—even wisdom as self-evident as "The world is full of greedy bottoms"—is a treasure.

Second, I do in fact hear from Danny Boy one last time, in a note that arrives a month or two after his six-month job has ended and he's traded weekend visits South for a full-time berth in MASTER Jeff's dungeon. The situation, it seems, hasn't really worked out and so, by mutual consent, Daniel has been emancipated, Glory Glory Hallelujah. In fact, in the meantime he's met another MASTER, one who lives right in San Francisco (though in a less-than-fashionable neighborhood), and *this* one, he realizes, is really The Real Thing, unlike now-I-can-see-how-inadequate-he-was Jeff. So he's moving to San Francisco to be a full-time slave, though to a part of the City, I note with relief, where I'm unlikely to run across him, in a slave collar, roaming the cereal aisle of Safeway.

And third, I have the ultimate Writer's Revenge. I write a short story about a thinly disguised Daniel in which—mea culpa—he gets killed off. And I sell the story. Three times.

It's a funny world. Months later I'm playing with a boy in his early 20s, a beefy switch and self-described vampire with a mean spanking stroke. When we've finished wrestling for top and we've both shot our versatile loads, we lie around talking, the way tricks often do.

"Total tops, utterly submissive bottoms—I know it must be a failing on my part," I say, "but I find it hard to take any of it seriously." And I tell him the condensed version of the Daniel story.

"That story reminds me," he says, "of this top I'd met, a guy who'd described himself as a tough, demanding Master. We played a few times, and then he asked me to be his full-time boy, which I had absolutely no interest in being. And damn if he didn't break down and start crying, telling me how much he loved me. It was so weird, I had to calm him down and baby him. Like there was a chance in hell I was gonna live with such a weirdo. He even lived in a dorky neighborhood, way out in the—"

"Um, what's his name?" I ask.

And Vampireboy tells me.

Life being chockablock with jaw-dropping O. Henry–type coincidences that any self-respecting author would shun, the top in question is, of course, Daniel's new MASTER.

And that's the very last I ever hear of slaveboy Daniel and his new MASTER. For all I know they're still together, blissfully, the owner and the owned. I hope so.

They're made for each other.

CHAPTER 13
Gender a-go-go: Transsexuals and Drag

I used to screw around with this cute, young, thoroughly smooth guy named Porter, who once showed up at my house carrying a brown paper bag. Partway through the petting process, he excused himself and vanished into the bathroom, little brown sack in tow. When he emerged a few minutes later, he was wearing a purple crushed-velvet miniskirt and elbow-length gloves. I was, well, taken aback. But after all, it was my pal Porter, whose hair reached halfway down his back and who was pretty enough to be a girl. I hitched his miniskirt up to his waist and gave him what he wanted; I'm no spoilsport. Still, as I pumped, I wondered if, even if I were into *women*, I'd want to have sex with the sort of woman who'd wear long black gloves and a purple velvet miniskirt to bed.

For a while I seemed to be a magnet for stealth drag queens. Popular culture—movies, TV shows, even rock songs—is full of ostensibly amusing plots where a guy brings home a girl only to discover "she" is really a man in a dress. I, on the other hand, was bringing home guy-type guys only to discover they were drag queens. I can never get anything right.

It's something of a pity, then, that I just don't find men in drag particularly sexy. Don't get me wrong—I'm not a misogynist, some of my best friends are transgendered, and I like femmy guys. Really I do. But the sight of a man in a dress just doesn't make Mr. Happy snap to attention. In bygone times, guys in drag were generally thought to appeal to suburban husbands with a bad case of the closets. In these queer-theoried days, though, we all know that gender, far from being a binary seesaw, is an overdetermined merry-go-round, a whirl of possibilities. So if guys in fishnet hose and Victoria's Secret teddies don't appeal to me, I'm clearly out of some loop or other. Maybe I'm dealing with issues of insecurity and self-image. Maybe it's internalized homophobia. Or maybe, tradition-bound fag that I am, I prefer my guys to be wearing pants. Whatever.

We're each and every one of us entitled to his turn-ons and, conversely, to letdowns as well. Having spent my formative years in a San Francisco crawling with drag queens both old-style, like dear Charles Pierce, and unconventional—the Cockettes, Angels of Light, Sisters of Perpetual Indulgence, and the whole gender-fuck crew—it's not that I'm nonplussed by guys who wander across the borderlines of sex. If anything, drag queens seem at this point in history (and I have the feeling it's the worst thing I could call them) banal. Some of my best friends are men who, at least sometimes, wear dresses. But, sorry, chicks with dicks never did it for me below the belt.

Porter's little costume change wasn't the only such surprise I've had. One night after the bars have closed, I meet a good-looking guy at Collingwood Park. It's nearly 3 by the time we get to his apartment, a crowded, funky little place in Hayes Valley. He puts a Prince album in the CD player and, before I can lay a hand on him, excuses himself to go to the bathroom.

Prince and I spend the better part of a half hour waiting for Barry to come out of the can. If it weren't the middle of the night, when other options are down to near zero, and if I hadn't followed this attractive guy all the way home, I might just leave him there in the bathroom and head out the door. But, I figure, what the hell. And besides, I like Prince.

When Barry emerges, he's wearing a floral print miniskirt, white stockings, a see-through plastic mac, and a wig that makes him look like the young Petula Clark. From head to toe—"toe" being white vinyl go-go boots and "head" being a thick layer of pancake makeup, false eyelashes, and more-than-ample applications of lip gloss—he's a near-perfect replica of the Carnaby Street birds I remember from my youth. Think Twiggy or Jean Shrimpton. He's even applied some faux-innocent cologne that smells just like the girls in my high school smelled. If I had any sort of learning curve at all post-Porter, I shouldn't have been blindsided. But somehow, I really hadn't anticipated spending the hours till dawn with a guy dressed as a Mod girl from swinging '60s London.

"Uh…" I start to say, but can't think of the words to follow that. (I suppose the appropriate thing would be, "Young lady, you march up to your room and wipe that makeup off your face. Now!")

"You like?" coos Barry.

I've been raised to have manners. "Um," I say, "it's something of a surprise, is all."

The CD player must be on auto-repeat, because I'm hearing the same Prince song for the second or third time. It's "Little Red Corvette," though if this were all a literary conceit, it would be "If I Was Your Girlfriend."

I think about walking out on Barry and his plastic mac. Really I do. But nobody likes to be a party pooper, especially not at 4 in the morning in a horny stranger's apartment. So, ever the perfect gentleman, I grit my teeth, gird my loins, and prepare to do the deed.

"Ready?" asks Miss Barry, somewhat incongruously.

"Ready," I say.

He bends over and hikes up his mini. He's wearing cute silken panties and garters, the stuff that makes straight guys get all wet, or so I hear, but the frilly gear doesn't do a thing for me. Still, his haunches are undeniably inviting.

"Pull them down, my panties down." Barry's voice has taken on a tone of hectoring urgency. *After all the trouble I've taken for you*, his subtext seems to say, *you can damn well jump-start me.* Prince's voice has shifted to falsetto. The evening is spinning rapidly out of control; nothing in my readings of gender theory has prepared me for quite this situation.

There are times in everyone's life, I guess, when caution is thrown to the winds and one chooses to launch oneself upon the Sea of Adventure, hoping one doesn't run aground on the Reef of Crap. So I pull down Barry's panties. Hey, he's inserted a perky little sex toy. The boy is full of surprises.

I reach over and turn off the damn CD player, reach for a condom, and try not to think of high school girls spraying on cheap cologne and applying lip gloss. As the saying goes, I would have closed my eyes and thought of England, but I was afraid I'd end up with a mental image of the young Marianne Faithfull being led away, naked beneath a fur blanket, at the infamous Mars Bar raid.

Out comes the dildo. In goes me. I can't say I'm at my shtupping best that morning, rating somewhere between "perfunctory" and "barely adequate." But I muddle through somehow. Marianne Faithfull would be proud. As I wobble out to the near-dawn streets and head for home I hum to myself. "As Tears Go By."

There were a couple of other times I played with guys in drag, most memorably with an Italian guy who was hairy, butch, built like a fireplug, and sounded like New Jersey every time he opened his mouth. He wanted, he said, to be my fucking slut. So the second or third time we played he gave me some money and I, ever the well-behaved top, left him loosely tied to the bed and went on a shopping trip. There is, in the heart of San Francisco's Latino neighborhood, amidst the bodegas and discount-shoe stores, a shop catering to the "larger woman," particularly the woman with 5 o'clock shadow and a penis. The spike-heeled shoes in extra-large sizes displayed outside the store looked like bargains, but once I got inside the prices shot up. It is not, I learned, so easy to buy black lace lingerie for husky Italian drag queens on a budget. I prowled through racks of false breasts and outfits that would make Frederick of Hollywood blanch. Bra, panties, garters, stockings, and I was on my way. When I rushed back to his place, Jerry was still in bed.

"You fucking slut," I growled. "I got you your fucking lingerie. All you do is lie in bed all day and expect me to buy you nice things. Is that it, you cunt?"

Jerry perked up considerably. I reached into my discreet little plastic shopping bag and brought out the frillies.

"Oh, please," he whimpered. "I'm such a fucking slut that I don't deserve them…but ple-e-ease…"

Suffice it to say that Jerry was no RuPaul. Once in drag, he looked like a butcher who'd been caught trying on his wife's unmentionables. But there was something about Jerry, with his muscles and coarse, black hair, wearing a cheesy bra and panties, fishnet hose pulled over his bulging calves, that was undeniably charming in a tawdry sort of way. Tied to his bed, stockinged legs spread, dick visible through black lace, he was every inch the cock-hungry bitch he claimed to be. But, let's face it, he wasn't about to star in *The Crying Game, Part 2*. There was no way in hell he could pass.

I did, however, like Jerry-cum-Geraldine. No problem fucking *him*. I was turned on by his thoroughly over-the-top transgressions, how sluttishly degraded he looked. What a fucking pussy. What a fucking cunt. When he played with gender, Jerry played hardball.

When it comes to gender theory and the labyrinthine transmutations of boys, girls, and others, I was, I'm afraid, rather a late bloomer. It's not that I had anything against transgendered people. It's just that, despite a growing barrage of tranny lit and tranny organizing, I couldn't figure out why some woman who used to be a man and now was a het housewife should share the podium at gay demonstrations. She could, after all, have been a plain old fag and let it go at that, without all the snipping and padding. I was, in a low-key way, cluelessly transphobic.

And then I met a man who used to be a woman, and all that changed.

He had a cute face, sometimes a scruffy beard, male pattern baldness, a nice hairy belly. And a vagina. We met because something in his online ad caught my eye. It's not that I'd been looking for a date with a female-to-male transsexual. Or even that I'd ever thought much about FTMs. There were those videos I'd seen at the queer film festival, that book by Loren Cameron. That was about it. But there was something about the ad that sucked me in, though to this day I'm not sure what.

We exchanged E-mail, talked by phone, he invited me over. Within a few minutes we were fucking. My penis was in his vagina. My dick in his pussy. I was 49 years old and I'd never touched a clit before in my life. It's not that I'm gynophobic; I'm just your basic Kinsey 5.9, about as homo as they come.

"A lot of us choose not to have surgery below the waist. Doesn't work so good, so I have the original equipment. Would you like a guided tour?" he asked before we actually got down to the deed.

"Sure," I said. He pulled down his underpants. I'd never been so close to labia before. And three things surprised me then, all at once: Even with a pussy, he was definitely a guy. None of this seemed even a little freakish. And my dick was rock-hard.

Well, I confess that it did freak me out a bit, back then, when he pulled off his T-shirt. There were scars from his "top surgery," the chest reduction. He told me he'd lost sensitivity there, so playing with his nipples didn't turn him on. Clearly, he'd given up a lot to get where he needed to go. But he seemed satisfied to be rid of it.

Before the change he'd been, I was taken somewhat aback to learn, a lesbian. A dyke with tits. A big ol' rugmuncher. And now he was a gay man with a receding hairline. He was "cute" rather than "butch." His voice was high-tenorish. But as my cock slid into his pussy, there was no doubt in my mind that I was fucking a man. Of *course* I was fucking a man—I'm gay, homos only get turned on by other guys, and I was turned on. Q.E.D.

Things in bed went fairly well. I chalked it up to beginner's luck and my knowledge of the feminist line on clitoral orgasms. I came. He came. I was, stupidly, a little proud of myself. I pulled the condom off and we lay in bed and talked for hours. Before the tranny boom I had assumed, in my superior way, that most transsexuals were closet cases whose internalized homophobia made them choose hormones rather than homosexuality. Lurking inside male-to-females, I figured, were oppressed fags who needed silicone boobs to give them permission to get it on with guys. And FTMs? Well, they were just bi women eager for a little male privilege. Or something like that.

But now here was this attractive man, this man I'd just had sex with, telling me he used to be a total dyke, a lesbian who, when she did do it with guys, generally did it for money. In fact, he'd been a pro domme, and, to hear him tell it, a rather nasty and successful one. So did the desire to become a man stem from internalized homophobia—or would that be internalized heterophobia? Unlikely—during and after the transition he continued to live with his girlfriend. They'd become a heterosexual couple. But then he came out. Again. Yet again. To himself and others. He'd become not just a man, but a gay man. He left his girlfriend and started sucking dick.

Whoa! I thought. I'd never been much of a queer essentialist, but here was this gay man telling me he'd used to be a lesbian, and I realized that the core of his identity wasn't gender-related but queerness-based. What mattered most wasn't the object-choice of his desires but their same-sex nature. *Whoa!* I thought. And then we had some tea.

That wasn't the last time I saw John. We got together occasionally over many months, more than a year, I think. I stopped shying away from his chest scars. I even went down on him, though I did, safely and tastefully, use a barrier. I began thinking of him, in my made-up politicalspeak, as a "differently abled fag." Did I wish he had a dick? Yeah, but not much.

Once when we went for a walk, we talked about the first time each of us had had sex. He told me about his countryside dalliance with a teenage boy. Afterwards I realized that all during John's story I'd been picturing two lads getting it on in a meadow. Things like that kept blowing me away.

He told me about the changes in his sexuality, how since he'd become a fag he'd gone from a lesbian-monogamous-nurturance mind-set to a desire to, well, trick. Back when he was a woman, he'd thought that gay promiscuity was typical male nastiness. Now he was gay himself, and he loved casual sex. Did the testosterone change him? Or did his new appearance give him permission to let loose his inner slut? Either way, it wasn't always easy for him to get laid. Some of the gay men he met eventually chickened out. But the more-or-less-het guys he met tended to be even worse, figuring they were chasing after novelty cunt but ending up with an actual guy instead. He'd pretty much given up on straight-identified guys, and I can't say I blame him.

A good friend of mine, kinky but thoroughly heterosexual, told me about three-way sex with a bi FTM and his girlfriend. "The only way I could stay interested in him was to think of him as a woman, a woman without tits." Sorry. I know the transboy in question; he's so obviously a man, a man without a dick. But a man. And it seems so unfair to overrule a person's entire being on the basis of the configuration of a few inches of flesh. I know that I wouldn't have thought this way a year or two ago, at least not so passionately. Sure, I knew some stuff about trannies, but all the theory in the world can't substitute for concrete experience, which in this case translates to "fucking."

Ongoing fucking. In the early days, the times after the first time, I was, shall we say, not immune to performance anxiety. Would the excitement remain after the novelty wore off? Was all this some worrisome harbinger of latent heterosexuality? And what was I doing diddling a clit, anyway?

Now the answer's pretty clear: I played with that clit because it belonged to a man who turned me on. He was good sex. *We* were good sex. We were gay sex.

It would be nice to report, fairy tales being what they are (and so many fairy tales being concerned with transformations of one sort or another), that our affair was an unqualified joy. It wasn't. It ended badly, and I found myself, in part, blaming John's willfulness. *Anyone who'd go to such lengths to become what he wanted to be, ruthlessly slicing off parts of his body and leaving them behind, probably has few qualms discarding buddies who don't, for one reason or another, measure up to his ideal.* As I thought that, part of me tut-tutted "Unfair! Unfair!" Nevertheless, I thought it.

Though things ended, and not well, I learned so much from him, so much. That gender is way mutable. That queerness is, at base, a lovely mystery. That it's never too late to broaden your horizons. That the brave and lucky among us can transmute themselves, never stop changing. And that eating pussy through Saran Wrap really sucks.

There's a coda to all this. A few months ago I met a couple of totally cute guys at a reading. A few weeks later I run into one of them at the supermarket; he's buying sherbet, I need milk. One thing leads to another. We end up in his car, out in the nighttime parking lot, making out furiously as the sherbet melts. OK, he's kind of short. His voice is kind of gender-indeterminate. He doesn't have much of a beard. Or an Adam's apple. And every time my hand creeps up his thigh, he firmly pushes it away. OK, OK, OK.

We finally cool down and make a date. Several days later I show up at his place, and within a minute flat we're sprawled, still clothed, on his bed. He looks up at me. Cute, so cute. Pretty, even.

"Um, I have something to tell you," he says.

I smile. "I'm not as stupid as I look. I know."

And this time, I knew just what to do with his clit.

CHAPTER 14
The Son Also Rises: Daddy/Boy Sex

The voice on the phone is soft-spoken, hesitant, as distant as Iowa. Which is, in fact, where he's calling from.

"Daddy?"

"Yes, son?"

"Oh Dad, I've missed you so much."

"I know you have, son, but I'm here now." I'm unzipping my fly. This is going to be good.

"I really need you, Daddy. I need your firm hand. See…I've been a…naughty boy."

My voice grows stern. This is, after all, why he contacted me online, asked to "do phone." Because he is indeed, at some level or other, a "naughty boy." So I say, "Well then, son, I'm going to have to do it. I'm going to have to get you across my knees and spank you."

"Ohhh, Daddy. I'm so sorry." There's a catch in his voice, like he's about to cry. My dick is way hard.

"Son, I'm going to have to discipline you." Should I do it? Should I bring on the special effects?

"Oh, no, please. I promise I'll behave."

All right, here come the sound effects. I hold the phone near my crotch and bring the palm of my loosely cupped hand down on my now-naked thigh a few times. I may not know very much about many things, but I do know how to spank so it sounds really loud.

I bring the phone back up to my mouth. "You promise to be good?"

"Oh yes, yes." I can hear the scared little boy in his voice, though he's in his early 30s.

I slap myself a few more times. Ow! That hurts. I decide to say it: "This hurts me more than it hurts you, boy." Which is the literal truth.

"Oh Daddy, I promise I'll be good. I promise to be a son any man would be proud of."

"I know you try, son." I use a tone that's indulgent, affectionate, but ruefully disappointed. "C'mere. Come sit on Daddy's lap. That's it. Throw your arms around me, boy."

"Oh, Daddy, your thing feels so big."

"Someday your penis will be this big."

"Re-e-eally?"

"Give Daddy a kiss." There's a slurping kind of sound from somewhere in the Midwest.

"Oh Daddy," the stranger says, "I love you so much."

"And I love you too, son."

I can't take it anymore. I shoot my load.

"Did you cum?" The voice on the phone has suddenly dropped an octave.

"Yeah."

There's the sound of heavy breathing, grunts. He comes, or at least makes sounds to make me think he's cum.

"That was great," I say. "Feel free to phone again."

The last thing he says before he hangs up is "I will."

As if.

Middle-aged geezers in search of smooth, young meat. Twenty-year-olds and 30-somethings looking for a good dirty time and maybe more. Daddies and boys. Where to begin?

"Daddy/boy" covers a lot of ground; there are as many modes of daddy/boy play as there are daddies and boys. My same-age primary partner and I call each other "Daddy" during moments of intense sexual surrender. A young guy I picked up on Castro Street was my "son" during an elaborate verbal incest fantasy we spun out during a long afternoon of otherwise vanilla sex. A pal of mine was legally adopted by his older boyfriend/daddy. And on and on. The roles of daddy and boy are, as they say in Theoryland, heavily overdetermined.

I realize I'm no big expert, just another middle-aged fag who loves being called "Daddy" while my often-but-not-always-much-younger boytrick is on his knees, on my dick, in my ropes, whatever. (And yes, I know there are "boys" in their 50s out there, as well as "daddies" barely old enough to vote, and more power to 'em. But I myself tend toward a more traditional age/role approach, OK?)

When I was a chronological boy, there was a paucity of visible daddy/boy stuff. (Or I willed myself not to see it. After all, I hung out in San Francisco's pre-epidemic leather bars but managed to remain blithely clueless about S/M practice. Of course, S/M culture was a lot less widespread then, but even so... Ah, callow youth!)

So why the daddy/boy thing? And why daddy/boy *now*? What accounts for its increasing visibility and popularity, its spiraling value as a currency of desire? Why did the last guy I had phone sex with start calling me "Daddy" before we even exchanged ages? (He turned out, in fact, to be 19 years younger, making the chronology just about right. Neat.)

My generation is the Stonewall generation, the first bunch of gay men to believe not only that we have a right to homosex but a right to homosex for the rest of our lives. Just as we get old enough to seriously lose status in the ultracommodified gay community, we go off and create a Daddy role for ourselves that allows us to remain objects of desire. Clever us.

Meanwhile, younger generations of gay men have for the last couple of decades been watching their elders drop like flies. If I were a young queer, I'd probably be pissed off because the virus-riddled Daddy Generation seems to be deserting the kids. Becoming a daddy's boy allows a young guy to search for a mentor both in and out of bed, to feel a continuity with a "community" that seems ever on the brink of vanishing yet is somehow able to renew itself. Intergenerational contact allows younger guys to hang onto us, in some sense to forgive us, and to help us carve out a space into which, with any luck, they'll one day mature. Daddyhood offers the promise that coming out does not doom one to extinction—sexually, emotionally, literally—at 35.

Daddy/boy play also gives bottomboys a commodity that remains a dirty little open secret: power from below. Even vanilla youth has its privileges, but this is particularly true in dominance/submission or S/M scenes. No matter how submissive a young guy may be, no matter how helpless within a scene, he always has an ace up his harness: He's younger.

You don't have to go to the gym to be "younger." You don't have to be smart or strong or even be good sex. You just have to have been born at the "right" time. No matter what else transpires, that power—the trump card of youth—remains real within the scenes dads and boys play out. At its best, that reserve of power allows a bottom to give himself permission to let go, to play deeper and harder. At its worst, it makes twinkies think they can jack some old geezer around and that the geezer will think, "Oh well, that's what a predatory old troll like me deserves" rather than "What a rude little asshole. Oh well, it's his fucking loss."

Oh yes, Dad gets good and tired of phone calls that aren't

returned, promises that aren't kept, plans that come to naught, the usual bullshit associated with self-absorbed, heartless kids. But on the other hand, daddyhood can work to empower aging tops, who are transformed from importunate old guys after young butt into something like the godhead. There's nothing better for one's self-image than realizing that you are indeed smarter, more mature, experienced, and talented—hell, that you're a better human being than you were when you were young. So the power thing can work both ways.

Daddy/boy also represents, in its charmingly paternal way, the return of traditional gender. In some queer quarters, unapologetic maleness is passé. Over in Postmodern Theoryland, gender is viewed as hopelessly old-fashioned and the drag queen is king. And meanwhile, in the Big Gay World, the hot commodity is identifiably male but not *too* butch. We like hairless bodies, we don't like male pattern baldness. We like lithe lads who are just barely postadolescent, not guys with beer guts. When you open up your copy of *Out*, all you see is beardless pretty boys who, even in leather drag, retain their androgynous aura. After a decade of stultifying sameness, though, the devalued has become fetishized, as is often the case. Bears growl that gut-is-good; gruff guys with facial hair have their own porn magazines. And daddies are desirable not despite but *because of* their secondary sexual characteristics. Daddies, like S/M tops, base their appeal on being Real Men, not deodorized, airbrushed little boys. Fetishized masculine signifiers can range from hairy backs to business suits, but the image is Traditional Male (whatever the reality may be). And that, it turns out, is what hardens some, maybe many, young cocks.

And softens hearts. The affection implicit in daddy/boy play gives it more potential for emotional vulnerability than other role-playing scenes: say, "master/slave" or "drill sergeant/recruit."

Sarge, after all, can't say "Hell, I love you, Private" while he's kicking butt. When it comes to tricks, affection can be the greatest taboo of all, but daddies and boys can play at love. Gnarly love, perhaps, but affection nonetheless. Before I shoot down a boy's throat, I love to tell him I'm feeding him the baby batter that created him. And when I spank him, I tell him it's "for his own good." Because it is.

The recent mainstreaming of kink has opened, as they say, a space in the discourse for all sorts of previously submerged stuff to flourish. In this post-postmodern age, transgression is in, and daddy/boy scenes sure can be taboo tramplers. Obviously, there's the suggestion of incestuous doings. A boy I played with quite awhile ago, handsome, hairy, and masculine, was the first guy I played with to use the *f* word. I had my dick up his ass when he said it: "Fuck me, Father." Father. *Father!* It was awesome, it was scary, and it made me want to pump even harder into my boy. I mean, "my son." But then there are endless opportunities for innovative nastiness within a scene. Daddy can be a submissive getting worked over by his strapping young son. Or Daddy's Little Boy can become Daddy's Little Girl. A 30-year-old businessman can play as a young kid. As long as the thought police don't find out.

Daddy/boy roles, like other kink-based binaries (top/bottom, sadist/masochist, whatever) add the heat of difference. Hets, of course, experience the tensions of gender all the time. But male/male sex, fraught with the dangers of hall-of-mirrors narcissism, can be jiggered so your partner is different but not *too* different. Unlike a woman, a man knows firsthand what other men really feel. But if the other man involved is older, younger, hairier, nastier, more submissive, it can make things all the more interesting.

Age gaps can be a big part of the kinky fun, but so can the intricacies of the mercy fuck. Many of us have learned that "lowering" ourselves to having sex with people we find unattractive, unworthy of us, or downright repulsive can add a lot of heat to a scene. And cute young men can find that giving it up for someone perhaps not so cute and definitely not so young makes for boundary-breaking fun. Older guys, on the other hand, can relax into chicken hawk status, finding a safe, legal, mutually satisfying way to make friends with their inner Dirty Old Man. But because the boy is looking for his daddy, Dad doesn't have to feel pathological or pathetic. (Though that can make for a hot scene as well, assuming the participants can handle it.)

For me, as I'm sure you've gathered by now, complexity is part of daddy/boy's appeal. Daddy/boy is a sexual scene that, more explicitly than most, plays with the basic building blocks of who we are and how we got that way. It's easy to see how even the most cursory of daddy/boy scenes, even just the use of the words, gets us in touch with some pretty deep shit.

There's an obvious place to start—the thoroughly ambivalent relationships most homos have with their own real fathers. The first porn story I ever wrote was a daddy/boy tale that made verbatim use of some of my childhood memories, only eroticized. My actual father is in many ways a stereotypical straight guy: a graceless emotional klutz, an armored personality seriously out of touch with himself. He's well-meaning, but every time he clumsily tells me he loves me, I wince. And for years he's looked like I might end up looking if I allow myself to get seriously out of shape, an unwelcome visible reminder that the rest of my life will be a physically downhill slide. But deep down, I want to be able to say "I love you too, Dad," and mean every word.

So when I become "Daddy," I try to be the father I wish I had: affectionate, demanding, worthy of respect. And hot. Like gay men everywhere, I've had to become my own father figure. When I play Daddy, I get to try my best. And my boys get to construct a new, improved model of their malehood, one which may include, paradoxically, a certain amount of punishment for the forbidden desire that brought them to me in the first place. It may sound pretentious, but it's true: When queer men play daddy/boy, we touch the deepest roots of our selfhood. Dad is both the first man we desire and the first man we betray. We want a dick just like the dick that hangs from dear old Dad. But in order to suck that dick, we become forever estranged from what Dad actually is: i.e., presumably straight. We're letting the Home Team down, walking away from our breeder birthright.

From Malcolm Forbes on his Harley to Archie Bunker in his armchair, men base identity on the trappings of power. (Even if, as it turned out, Forbes was quite queer.) Too many het guys base entirely too much of their identities on the power perks of being a straight male. It is, like being white in a racist culture, the Great Fallback Position. A guy can be out of work, undereducated, unattractive, divorced, whatever, but at least he ain't one of them fags. Having a dick is what gives him power, and by damn, he knows where to put it.

Sonny boy turning out to be queer is not only perceived as disobedience but as ingratitude. It doesn't even matter, it seems, if he carries on the genetic line as part of the queer parenting boom; no gay male book is more vilified by homophobes than *Daddy's Roommate*. So, clearly, growing up gay, with its awful secret of compromised maleness, makes probably all us queer guys both rebellious and ashamed.

When Daddy plays with a boy, a son, a pussyboy, he's asserting his own "genuine masculinity." He may be a homo, but he's availing himself of a number of patriarchal perks. The male power position is his. Cute boy equals the trophy wife. It may all be rather problematical, politically speaking, but Christ, life is hard, and we're entitled to some fun. Three cheers for dick!

Of course, Daddy's maleness is not only a threat; it's catnip too. It carries a potent erotic charge that can never quite be simply, safely resolved. Daddy/boy desire is so damn fraught because it's so much like real life. Only more so. Even the most abusive-seeming of scenes can be touched by mutual affection and respect. And even the most unequivocal declarations of love are informed and transformed by power relationships. (Oh, *père* Foucault!)

It would be comfortably neat, in a vulgar Freudian way, if the boys involved in daddy/boy play had histories of insufficient fathering. But in my informal, hands-on, pants-down research, that's simply not true. Some had distant or absent fathers, others report extraordinarily close relationships with their dads, and many had experiences somewhere in between. It would seem that the tangled skein of maleness, homosexuality, and the erotic is extraordinarily complicated, which is what makes it so damn interesting and hot.

We're not dealing just with unresolved personal issues here; we're dealing, damn it, with archetypes. At the risk of seeming hopelessly pretentious, a risk I've run before and will no doubt run again, daddy/boy sex is a spiritual quest. The specifics may vary, but some common themes emerge.

A boy is a seeker, looking for that powerful figure who both disciplines and nurtures, whose hands can bestow love or punishment, who ultimately can take his boy up in his strong arms and bring him love and joy and peace. Surrender, transcendence, and bliss.

Sound familiar? Yes, guys, it's the religious quest, more specifically the monotheistic quest, and most specifically, the Christian paradigm. Our Father might hang out in Heaven, but it's a bit easier to find him when he's in the bedroom. In most daddy/boy scenes, Dad's the dominant one, the powerful one, the Lord. There are flips, to be sure—scenes in which a younger guy tops an older—but they're the exception, not the rule. But just what does the hardworking dad get out of all this?

The short answer is: power. But is it as simple as that? Does God, after all, really have fun ruling the Universe? Seems doubtful. There's the responsibility of looking after his unruly children, of having to keep the cosmos spinning, having to clean up the mess every time one of his offspring fucks up. The exercise of unlimited power must be no picnic. No wonder He gets cheesed off every once in a while and sends earthquakes and tornadoes and things.

The gay daddy, like Jehovah, has all the problems of the diligent top. He has at least the theoretical responsibility of keeping the scene going. He's responsible for both his boy's well-being and his own. He's the one to bring his boy to tears and the one to wipe those tears away. Yes, yes, he's worshiped and obeyed, but surely there are easier ways to get sucked off.

Like any good deity, a good daddy needs empathy. Patience when his lad goes astray, as go astray he surely shall. And no expectation that the world he's created will proceed exactly as planned. Bad daddies, like Wotan in *The Ring* operas, can fuck their boys over, and, just as important, can fuck themselves up as well. But good daddies, the best daddies, transmute time, mortality, and need into something that can pass for sacred. And get their heavenly rocks off too.

EVEN DADDIES NEED DADDIES, reads the T-shirt my partner gave me. And yeah, that seems to be true. So when I first played with my German top, Herr Vater, the handsome middle-aged sadist, I knew I'd found someone I'd let see my little boy, my kinky inner child.

I found myself apologizing to him, to my Master, my Papa. Not *pretending* to apologize, which is quite another matter. Truly, from some deep part of my gut, sobs of grief-stricken remorse arose. I begged His pardon for all my bad ways, for my being a pervert pig and a bad boy. For my failure, for my sin, for my very existence.

"Oh, Daddy Sir. I'm so sorry, so fucking sorry, so fucking sorry, Sir."

Not once did I think about how silly I might have looked, how theatrical the whole thing was. The word *inauthentic* never crossed my mind. I *was* the bad little son, groveling with a hard-on, and my stern father was sorrowfully but necessarily teaching me the meaning of good and evil.

Whack! The riding crop—*my* riding crop—came down hard upon my thighs; searing pain that I usually can't take, don't enjoy. But now it was better than I deserved, and I drank in every stroke.

When I looked up into his stern gray eyes, I was cocooned in a theology of suffering. All the pain, loss, disappointment of the world, of mortality, was distilled into the stroke of the crop.

Oh fuck.

Herr Vater is damn near perfect, at least for me. I've learned, from below, a lot about scenes from him. No, his monologue has scarcely been inventive, just the same few phrases over and over interspersed with "You're a bad boy, aren't you?" which I dutiful-ly answer in the affirmative each and every time. But the repeti-tion, far from constraining the scene, opens it out, nearly hyp-notically. My superego goes on autopilot, and the faggot kid in me can play. *Will* play, damn it! Never mind that the game con-sists of confessing every vulnerability, each failing, every unspoken trespass I've ever committed. Never mind that the game is really about the strangeness of existence, about good and evil, about guilt beyond forgiveness. It's the only game in town, and if the odds are overwhelmingly with the house, well fuck it, I'll play anyway.

So clearly, there's a cosmic dimension to all this, and it's not just about Daddy, it's about Big-Dicked God. Agreed? Well, yeah, but then all sex is about God when you get right down to it. Religion and cock sucking are the two great occasions for getting down on your knees. Because the greatest conundrum we puny li'l humans face is the mystery of self. We're flesh bags dubiously blessed with self-consciousness. We're given all this freedom, the big existential hoo-ha, and yet we're ultimately the slaves of our bodies, which is to say time, which is to say entropy, which is to say Death. Bummer, huh?

Heterosexuality seems to provide a detour from dying: kids. Maybe *we* won't always be sitting there watching reruns of *The Brady Bunch* on Nick at Nite, but our progeny will, carrying bits of our genetic soup into the far-flung future. Well, not *your* DNA, not if you're like most queer men. Yes, yes, there's Heather and her two Mommies, and the boom in queer child-rearing is certainly to be respected. (It's only when breeding's privileged— "See, we fags can be unselfish too. Some of us are even raising kids, *just like normal people*"—that it becomes more than a little queasy-making.) But the idea that homos are childishly narcissistic because we choose not to jam the already crowded planet with little reproductions of ourselves, well...

We labor under the illusion that we're in control of our lives because anything else would be just too scary. It's hardly any wonder that queers are, at least reputedly, overrepresented in the creative arts. It's another route to immortality, and yes, I'd be pleased as punch if, a millennium hence, some fag Jetson ran across an antique digital copy of *Kinkorama,* even if futurefag ended up laughing hysterically over its outdated prose and even more outdated notions of desire.

There was this cute Las Vegas boy I met online: 28, beautiful, into being abused by hairy old men. Hairy old me. "I love being degraded by dirty old men," he tells me, and my penis does a little jig.

"Can I ask," I type out, somewhat hesitantly, "why you want that?"

Pause. He's not an airhead; it's a hard question.

"I don't know," he finally types out, "I guess it has to do with my real father." Well, of course it does. I keep picturing him naked as I spit on him, slap him around—in his words, "fuck him up." I want to erase the line between degradation and ennoblement, pleasure and its opposite, youth and age—ultimately, me and him. At least temporarily. Clearly, I think too much.

We chat for a long while, spiraling down to dark fantasies of humiliation and pain. At one point, he asks me, and it's a fair question, why I want to abuse young bottomboys like him.

"Maybe several reasons," I type back. "Because you want it, for one. And because the bond that can occur between a dad top and a boy bottom can be amazing and beautiful. And, to tell the truth, because you're young and beautiful, and that gives you a power I both crave and resent, and part of me wants to punish you for the desire I have for you."

This was, pretty clearly, a bit much for a brand-new online acquaintance, but the boy seemed to understand, to take it in stride, even to be excited by it. We typed back and forth for another half hour or so. I told him I was going to be in Las Vegas soon. He told me how much he wanted to be degraded and abused by me. I suggested he phone me, a marker, though far from an infallible one, of his sincerity. He leapt at the opportunity, and within a minute my phone rang.

The connection was awful, but I liked his voice, what I could discern of it between bursts of cell phone static. And we were off to the archetypal races, the familiar dance of Daddy, loving yet strict, and his boy—desirable, desired, disappointing, dirty, the fagboy who let Dad down.

It didn't take me too long to cum.

It's all so deep, so dark, so damn much fun. But one nagging question: By replaying the tapes of our childhood needs, by remixing them, do we make ourselves freer, happier? Or do we simply reinforce the most neurotic, dysfunctional parts of our lives? When I beat that artist till he begged me not to stop but to beat him more and more until he couldn't help but shoot his load, I mean, what was happening there? Catharsis? Or really sick shit? But then, what's happening during any sex, particularly homosex? It is, as Scott O'Hara said, "rarely pure and never simple."

Being Daddy's not just a kink, it's an adventure. I've lost my heart to cute boys who flirt and encourage pursuit, then run off to their rooms to play with their little friends. I've snagged the hearts of other boys, for an hour or for years. I've become the man I've always wanted to be. I've realized that part of me will always be a child. I've learned a lot. I've kissed some beautiful faces. And whipped some beautiful butt. And I got my rocks off in the process. What more could an aging sex fiend hope for?

CHAPTER 15
Lie Down With Speed Freaks, Get Up With No Sleep: Drugs and Need

I'm a sucker for Boys With Problems. Unsurprisingly, I guess, that's gotten me into trouble. Trouble like Corey.

Late one night I'm tense, pissed off, and horny. I'd been stood up for a date, had gotten a parking ticket in the process, and a drunk in an SUV had almost killed me on my way home. I've slunk into the last refuge of late-night losers, the AOL chat rooms. I'm halfheartedly cruising when I get an Instant Message from someone whose screen name promises he'll be a great daddy's boy, and his subsequently E-mailed picture makes my perverted old heart skip a few beats. He is, without a doubt, the boy of my dreams, or at least the next-best thing. And he doesn't even want to see my pic.

After 2 A.M. the odds are good that a sizable proportion of online cruisers are tweaked out of their brains on crystal meth. So when my "Are you partying?" brings a "Yes," I'm hardly surprised. Or deterred. We talk by phone, and he seems perfectly sweet, if a bit sketchy. And his place is just a short middle-of-the-night motorcycle ride away. I hope that the drunk in the SUV either is safely off the roads by now or has driven over a cliff.

When I pull up at Corey's house sometime after 3, he's waiting outside: tall, thin, bleached blond, and jaw-droppingly cute. It's one of those "Jesus, I'm out of my league" moments. But when I take my helmet off, he doesn't flinch. Better: He says,

"Wow, you're really hot." *There IS a God*, I'm thinking.

I'm semi-used to dealing with guys on speed, and as guys on speed go, he seems to be midway on the Tweak-o-Meter. He takes me upstairs to his apartment. "Quiet. My roommate's asleep," Corey whispers as we creep into his room. Well, *creep* is perhaps the wrong word: His small room is so cluttered with piles of dirty clothes that it's impossible to find a square foot of floor across which to creep. Luckily—and here I break my mother's heart—I get off on messy, really messy, rooms. By now my dick is firing on all cylinders.

"God," says the pretty, tweaked-out boy, "you're so my type." This is thoroughly convenient, since he's mine as well.

I'm not sure when I started to fixate on skinny boys in their 20s. And I'm not sure just what that signifies, though I have a few clues. I used to frame my attraction in generalized daddy/boy terms, then focused in on scrawny boys' apparent physical vulnerability, but eventually came round to wondering if it might not have something to do with one of my very first full-bore crushes, a gawky, skinny boy named Andy with whom I played chess back in high school. At least I think he was skinny and gawky. This all took place long, long ago and memory is supremely unreliable, but I do remember him as being nerdy and very thin, and that's exactly the point. Andy and I never did anything, not even remotely, though my teenage hormones were on a constant tear, and I find it novelistic—and oddly pleasing—to think my late-middle-age sexuality is trying to resolve unfulfilled desires hatched so very long ago.

Whatever the case, however murkily insoluble the mysteries of lust may be, it's immensely gratifying when Corey plunks himself down on his disheveled bed, glances at me through pupils big as pie plates, says "God, I'm so horny," and pulls his dick out. His cock is lovely, medium-size, and, judging from its reddened complexion, has lately seen a lot of use. Corey loses no time slipping off to Masturbationland, working with a steady, full-hand approach. Not knowing quite what to do, afraid that this apparition of totally fucked-up loveliness will vanish without a trace like some Cinderella on meth, I pull my own cock out and kneel on one of the few bits of accessible floor in his vicinity. His hand comes away from his cock. My mouth takes its place. His dick tastes of youth, speed, and Vaseline.

Some guys when their cocks are being sucked lean back in a do-me posture and wait to be pleasured. Others will stroke your hair, your face, reach down for your nipples, your cock. Corey is one of the latter. "Mmm," he mumbles, "that feels so fucking good." That makes me feel good as well; making beautiful men feel pleasure is a privilege not to be taken lightly. I slide a hand beneath his not-very-clean T-shirt. Pay dirt. Corey has the hairless, slightly sunken chest of a 14-year-old. Not just any 14-year-old but one who forged notes from his Mom so he could get out of gym class. I am, I'm terrifically grateful to note, not even remotely into actual underage boys—to me, even a 19-year-old seems like jailbait, chronological sin with a penis. But that look, the scrawny look of the kid but on a man-boy in his 20s, that's the look makes my heart leap and my dick drip. My dick is dripping now.

"Hey," he says, "you want a bump of crystal?"

I take my mouth off him just long enough to decline with what I hope sounds like a polite, nonjudgmental "No thanks."

Corey is, physically, pretty much exactly my dreamboy. The blandly handsome face of a choirboy gone to seed. An impossibly lean body. A dick that, despite crystal, has no problem staying hard in my mouth. And, miraculously, the attraction is mutual. He proves it by tugging my shirt off, then maneuvering us both around until his mouth gulps down my cock. For a 3 A.M. AOL date, this is going very well indeed.

His mouth leaves my dick. "I'm going to do another bump," he says. "Sure you don't want any?"

"Nope," I reply. "Take your shirt off."

As he bends over the room's only table, snuffling speed off a tabletop littered with CDs and bits of paper scrawled with men's phone numbers—including mine—my eyes gulp down his torso, rail-thin. There's something indescribably evil about watching this beautiful, slightly ravaged boy abusing drugs as I sit there stroking my cock. It's not quite Dennis Cooper territory, but it's in the neighborhood.

Crystal methamphetamine is a very discursive drug, so we talk for a while, stroking sometimes our own, sometimes each other's cocks. I can't get enough of watching Corey's pretty mouth move as speaks, quietly but with a chemical urgency. He comes from New York, he says, from money, the Upper East Side, he's lost his boyfriend to an ugly breakup, his best friend to AIDS, left a good job to move West. He's been in San Francisco for a couple of years, getting progressively more fucked-up on meth. He wants to get clean. He's been awake for over three days.

Oh, and one other thing. He's really into older guys only, but a lot of them have kept chasing him, wouldn't let him be. He shows me a note, a pleading, semi-pitiful note one of his pursuers has sent him. This is not only massively indiscreet (though I do, mea culpa, read the entire note), it also puts me in an odd position, one I immediately recognize. Danger bells clang, yellow warning lights flash. If I behave myself, I can join the ranks of Corey's admirers. If I don't, I'll be placed on the list of predatory old creeps and someday Corey will be telling another one of his tricks about *me*.

Corey does another line of speed. Crystal provides an oddly paradoxical sex high. On the one hand, it makes the tweaker feel invulnerable, ready to go way past his normal limits. On the other, it typically makes for at least some degree of impotence, not to mention paranoia, sketchiness, and a general inability to keep things together.

Once, for instance, I went over to an orgy at a guy's apartment, bringing some rope as requested. I got there to discover six or eight guys, all naked, all tweaked, some shooting up. It was pretty much a lower-depths kind of thing, and if I'd had less of a sense of adventure and more common sense, I would have turned tail and gotten the hell out of there right away. Instead, I soon was serving as Bondage Master to the tweakers, tying one naked guy up and holding him down as another guy injected him with meth. I was working away at my square knots while the drug abuse loped on, William S. Burroughs as Eagle Scout.

I was the only sober guy there, so my top powers were intact whilst all around me guys were slamming crystal into their own and each others' veins. But the glow of my power wore off quickly. When I went to the bathroom and caught sight of myself in the mirror, a mirror above a counter strewn with used hypodermic points and empty glassine envelopes, I decided enough was enough. Rescuing my ropes, I left the apartment as graciously as possible while the drug-soaked little orgy raged on, its participants increasingly, obviously edgy.

As fate would have it, a few days later I ran into one of the speed freaks I'd tied up, a pleasant-looking fellow with a brush cut and some missing teeth. He told me that shortly after I'd left, things had spun rapidly out of control. Somebody's wallet went missing, accusations were flung, clothes were tossed out the window into the street below, eventually the cops were called. I wasn't even a little bit sorry I'd left when I did.

Corey told me early on that he used speed to get over his sexual hang-ups, that he never messed around without it. When I first looked at Corey, all I saw was the boy of my dreams, and therefore an automatic sex machine. So when I realized how fucked up, and therefore vulnerable, he was, I felt an onrush of power, beneficent power perhaps. I was in fact so much more together than this immensely desirable kid. I was too smart to think I could save him from drugs, himself, or much of anything else, but I found myself nevertheless in the by-now familiar dual position of Nurturing Dad and Predatory Old Man. It may not be a particularly comfortable place to be, but it sure as hell is an interesting one.

Somewhere around 4 or 5 in the morning, Corey sucks up the last line. Time to go out and score some more meth.

"At this hour?" I ask.

"We're talking about speed," he says.

"Good point."

"Can I wear your chaps?" he asks.

"No, I don't think so."

"How about your jacket?"

Well, it is cold out, and I figure it's a matter of trust; if he's going to leave me untended in his apartment, it would be rude not to let him borrow my leather jacket, right?

He's dialing his phone. "I'm calling my dealer."

A terse phone conversation, which I try not to listen to, ensues. Corey hangs up and says, "He's meeting me a few blocks away. I should only be gone a half hour."

"OK, you can wear the jacket." While he's been on the phone, I've fished my keys out of the pocket.

"Thanks a lot." He's so cute, so sexy, such a religious experience when he smiles his drugged-out little smile.

Two hours later, he and my jacket still haven't returned. Not for the first time in my life, I find myself wondering *What the fuck am I doing here?* Drifting in and out of sleep, I curse myself for lending him my jacket, thereby precluding an easy escape. I'm trying to get some sleep, fighting the springs on Corey's broken-down mattress, when there's a knock at the bedroom door.

It's a boy who tells me he's crashing at Corey's. Jamie has magenta hair, nails bitten down to the quick, and is on the smelly side, a thoroughly dissipated-looking lad. Needless to say, I'm captivated.

He says he's the pal of the dealer Corey has gone to score from, and he's worried. He was expecting Corey to meet him and Aaron hours before, but Corey never showed. *Fuck*, I think. *My fucking jacket!*

We chat aimlessly for a while, keeping an increasingly anxious vigil for my missing trick. Every noise brings tweaked-out Jamie to the window, now lit up by dawn. I watch his every wired move, wondering, wondering…

"Hey, how old are you?" I ask at last.

"Nineteen." Legal.

"Can I suck your cock?"

He doesn't say anything. He just unzips his fly and lies back. The world outside Corey's window is wide-awake and facing the new day.

After I've sucked off Jamie's skinny, funky dick, after he's jacked me off, after I've finally resigned myself to riding home, freezing, in my shirtsleeves and praying I'd recover my leathers at a later date, the phone rings. It's Corey. He's gone to where the dealer had said he'd be, he waited there, then went looking for him, then the police had stopped him, then he ran into friends of his, then… Whatever. Speed freaks. Jesus!

"See you in five minutes," Corey says.

He shows up an hour later. He is, thank God, still wearing my jacket. I'm once again surprised by how sexy he is, in that wasted way of his. Jamie says hi, then pads off to the living room. Corey shuts the door, pulls his dick out, and, without a word of explanation or apology, starts jacking off. I get down on my knees and start sucking his half-hard dick. What else can I do? He looks so beautiful.

"Jamie's a trip," he says.

"Mmm," I agree, my mouth full of Corey.

"He been here long?"

"Mmm," I say.

"He's, like, Aaron's partner. Aaron's the dealer I went looking for."

"Mmm," I reply.

"Jamie didn't get on your nerves?"

"Mmm," I demur.

"Um, you and him…"

"Mmm?"

"Did you guys mess around?"

"Mmm-hmm." I see no reason to lie, even gutturally.

"Weird…he usually only goes for black kids who are younger than he is…Hey, would you reach over and hand me that pipe? There may still be some crystal in it."

And so I kneel there, amidst piles of smelly clothes, sucking the cock of an unbelievably attractive boy while he smokes an early-morning hit of speed. It is, verily, a decadent moment, one fraught with weighty moral questions. Am I somehow complicit in his drug use? If I weren't there, wouldn't another old guy, one most likely not as caring and safe, be in my place? Or is that just a rationalization provided by my hard dick? And to what depths could I happily sink in my pursuit of this thin, handsome tweaker? I push his legs up so I can access his asshole, say a silent prayer to the goddess of dysentery, and plunge my tongue into his insides. But, though I want to rim him forever, the long, long night is catching up with me. I flop onto the unmade, junky bed and watch as he jacks off and jacks off and jacks off and finally comes. Somewhere along the line I've cum too, and without much ceremony I zip up and get ready to leave.

"My roommate's awake," Corey says.

"Yes?"

"He's a gay Catholic priest. Lapsed. He's OK."

And sure enough, as we walk to the front door, there's Father Whoever, sitting at the computer, his bulky body bare-naked, a little ponytail down his neck. I'm in no shape to introduce myself, but I do think the priest part is a nice touch, the sort of thing that would seem too contrived if I put it in a short story. Corey and I hug and dry-kiss—he has crystal mouth—and I wobble off to my motorcycle, riding home through streets full of responsible folks heading off to work.

Over the succeeding weeks I obsess about Corey, phone and leave messages for him, and every so often those messages get returned. Sometimes, usually in the wee hours, he calls and wants to know if I'd come over. But mostly I see him online, usually after 1 or 2 in the morning. Every once in a while I get to actually head across town and spend some time with him, bringing along my chaps so he can dress up in Daddy's clothes. Corey is, of course, always on drugs. Speed, yes, but also X, GHB, K, a whole alphabet soup of postmodern pharmaceuticals. The thing about folks with heavy drug habits is that all their needs seem to have boiled down to A Single Need and, without getting moralistic about it, the need to ingest one substance or another seems to me to be a lot more boring than the richly textured, endlessly twisted needs of sexual desire. If I'm going to be addicted to something, I'd rather it was flesh than some powder in a little plastic bag.

OK, maybe Corey is the sort of boy I should have walked away from posthaste. But, beyond his Germanically handsome young face and his pale, thin body, there is also something genuinely likable about him, peeking out through his sketchy speed-freak fucked-upness.

His story is always the same: He hasn't been using much speed lately, he's been cutting back, this is a rare exception, he's fallen in with a bad crowd, he wants to go back to New York, maybe, and get his life together. At the beginning I wanted to believe his almost-every word, I wanted to help him, provide support while his so-called friends were busy mistreating him, ripping him off, leading him further into the morass of crystal use. Eventually, though, I settle for lying beside him with my hand on his prominent ribs, feeling his skinny chest vibrate as he tells his tales of woe. It's not even that the sex is particularly good. It's not. He's not even into kink, not at all really, though he obligingly lets me slap him around a bit. But basically he likes having his cock sucked, he likes sucking my dick, and our sessions usually conclude with him incessantly whipping his speed-limpish dick into a froth. I can live with that.

Still, there are moments, lovely moments, when we seem to connect, when there's at least the appearance of tenderness, when he opens his parched lips and l stick my tongue down his throat and make him moan. There are moments when I feel splendid about making such a drug-hazed, emotionally needy, beautiful, fucked-up kid feel "good," not just "used." Or so I want to believe.

One day Corey phones me and invites me over. He's been up for a few days, has done some ecstasy, really wants to see me, really wants to "try some stuff out." And when I obligingly arrive at his squalid apartment, it does seem that he's in a new mood: more centered, more giving, more passionate.

I let him put on my chaps. It always takes a good deal of cajoling to get him naked underneath; he hates to take his pants off during sex, and his jack-off sessions are almost always conducted with his boyish dick protruding cutely from his fly. It seems an apt metaphor for something he's told me: Despite his cute slacker looks and demeanor, he'd had a rather rigid upbringing, was sexually repressed, and uses speed in order to let down his guard enough to enjoy sex at all. He's in therapy, he's on meds, but clearly This Boy Has Issues. *Of course. Otherwise,* I whisper to myself, *why would he be having sex with me at all?*

This time I've brought my toy bag and my digital camera. I tie up his dick and take a picture. I flog him lightly and take pictures of his reddened back and butt. I take pictures of him sucking my dick, and when late in the afternoon I piss on him, I juggle the camera and take a picture while the warm stream hits his pale, narrow chest and runs down his fat-free belly. And then we lie around for hours, Corey snorting an occasional bump of speed, and talk and talk. He tells me more about his past, the time he's spent in Amsterdam, the rich Dutch man who still wants to take him back to Europe. And we talk about the future, the first time we have, about what we could do on future get-togethers. Is any of this true? Does it matter? This time when I leave the apartment, I feel less like a slightly pathetic old guy hung up on a beautiful youth and more like a man who's found a friend. A much younger friend, a friend with problems, but a friend nonetheless.

Just a few days later, all that gets cast into doubt. I'm online late at night when Corey's screen name pops up on my Buddy List. I send him an Instant Message: "Hey. I had a great time Monday."

"Monday?"

"Yeah, when I was over at your place," I type back.

"You were?"

Christ on a bicycle! I know Corey is always fucked-up on drugs, but this is absurd. I thought we'd gotten closer than ever before, but the kid had been entirely absent. Fuck.

"Corey, I have the pictures to prove it."

"Send them to me."

"I'll send one."

And I do, a picture of him bare-chested, Daddy's black leather jacket hanging from his skinny frame, his dick and balls, as usual sticking out of his open jeans but this time all tied up.

When he's downloaded the JPEG he asks, "How many did you take?"

"About a dozen. You don't remember?"

"Send me the rest."

"Fuck, you don't even remember what happened."

"I let you take them, didn't I? Not sending them is like stealing from me."

As pissed off as I am, I've already decided to send them all, so after a bit more bickering I E-mail them, all but one, my favorite—the one showing his lean, pale body entirely naked for once, dick in hand, looking thoroughly handsome. And then I go to bed, pondering the twists and turns of obsessive lust.

I decide to let Corey make the next move. It's tough, though. The more I've gotten to know Corey, the more unsuitable an object of desire he's seemed. And the more fiercely I've wanted him.

A few days later I'm online when Corey IMs me.

"I'm at this guy's house, and he wants a third. Want to come over?"

I don't, not really. I want to play with Corey all by myself. But I'm horny, he's not always so accessible, so I figure *What the hell?*

"Sure. It's all right with him?"

"Yeah. He's kind of a dork. He'll do whatever we say."

Half an hour later I'm in an expensively furnished apartment, hanging with Corey and his host: a pudgy, rather plain-looking man in his late 30s.

"You want to fuck him?" Corey asks.

I don't want to, not at all, but I do know how to be a good guest. I plow the man, Allen, doggy-style for a bit, always keeping one eye on Corey's jacking-off. I pull out of Allen's loose ass and Corey takes over. It becomes rapidly evident that both Corey and Allen are very, very stoned: GHB and speed, as it turns out, with a chaser of Viagra that's keeping Corey harder than I've ever seen him before.

"Want some?"

"No thanks," I say, and I don't.

After an awkward while, Corey starts sucking my cock. Allen crouches down with a digital camera, acting a little weird.

"No pictures," says Corey, but Allen snaps away anyway, then suddenly starts groaning, stands up, and leaves the room. I shoot my load into Corey's lovely mouth.

Allen returns, testy. "That GHB made me sick. You guys didn't care at all, did you?" There's a nasty edge to his voice.

God, I think, *the weird places my dick has gotten me.*

I figure it's time to go. I pull my clothes on while the drug-soaked duo bicker, then thank Allen for his hospitality (such as it was) and show myself out the door.

A day or two later the phone rings. Corey. "Allen is really tripping, man. It's scary."

"Huh?"

"The other night, when you sent me pictures? That wasn't me online. Allen hacked into my AOL account and was posing as me. That's how he found out about you. That's why he wanted me to invite you over. Now he's saying horrible things about you. And he's threatening to send those photos you took to my family."

"And you invited me over there to meet this psycho?"

"I didn't know about it, I swear." He sounds pretty tense. And tweaked.

I begin to panic. For all my trolling about amidst the lower depths—all the risky, stupid, humiliating things I've done in pursuit of sex—I've actually come out fairly clean. At least one friend of mine was murdered by a trick—it's a dangerous world—but the biggest problems I've had lately have been a stubborn case of venereal warts and where to put the bottle of poppers my latest conquest has left behind. Suddenly, though, my comfy little cocoon is shattered.

Weeks before, in a postcoital moment, Corey had told me stories of the tweaker demimonde; how evil leather queens invited boys back to their place and shot them full of witches' brews of drugs, often having unprotected sex with their unconscious bodies. At the time I'd thought it all sounded just too Dennis Cooper for words. Now I myself have come face-to-face with a drug-soaked monster. More: I've called home from his place, and if he hit redial, he could have gotten my phone number from my outgoing message. He has, literally, my number.

"Hang on," I say, "I'll be right over."

Corey has often looked what I liked to think of as "elegantly wasted." This time, though, he looks just plain wasted, dark-gray circles ringing his pale eyes.

"I'm really freaked," he says. "Allen's been stalking me. He turns up here at 4 in the morning and demands to be let in. He's said he'll send those pictures to everyone on my E-mail list. And he's been saying awful things about you."

I hold Corey's hands—his pale, slim, beautiful hands—and try to get rational. What to do? Tell the cops? That would just infuriate the loony, should he find out, and anyway we have no proof of his threats. Do nothing? Corey assures me that Allen's obsessions know no bounds.

The phone rings.

"I bet it's Allen," Corey says. We ignore it.

While Corey's becoming calmer, I'm growing more alarmed. At the very least, I'll have to change my AOL passwords. At the most, my partner and I will be haunted by mysterious midnight calls and FedExed dead animals. But, I have to remind myself, I really have only Corey's word on all this and, let's face it, his grasp on reality can be a bit tenuous, no matter how fucking cute he is.

Then the door opens. It's Father Bill, and he's looking distraught. "Why didn't you answer the phone? I was worried that something had happened." And yes, Corey's roommate confirms, everything about Allen is true. He's been showing up at all hours, throwing stones at the windows of the apartment, even camping out on the front stairs. More than once Father Bill has had to threaten to call the cops before the weirdo would go home.

The three of us go around in circles till there's no more to be said. So I head for home, feeling slightly guilty because I've found Corey's panicked vulnerability so damn sexy.

As the days pass, punctuated by phone updates about Allen's continued bad behavior, I want to hate Allen, I really do. Bad. But, damn it, I can see where he's coming from. He has this enormous, unmanageable, drug-fueled crush on this boy who doesn't give a shit about him. And though I've never misbehaved the way Allen has, I can remember hanging out around an aerobics studio in hopes of seeing a boy I had a big crush on, detouring to walk past his apartment building and having my heart leap because the object of my lust lived there. Given more desperation, less maturity, evil drugs, who knows what sleazy things I might be capable of?

Fortunately, Allen's bile never results in any moves against me. No midnight phone calls, no weird E-mail. Nothing. But my relationship with Corey, never on the firmest of foundations, has narrowed down to What to Do About Allen. No more sex. No more of anything except Corey's drama, in which, I figure, I've gone from having a bit part to being a supporting player. Corey, though, even more self-absorbed than ever, is treating me like I'm his audience.

The kid has gone from being Charmingly Fucked-up to just plain fucked up. He's always seemed fragile, with his pale skin, bony body, fine-featured face. Now he's coming apart at the beautiful seams. He's 26, and his life's falling apart. Falling apart is what your life is supposed to do when you're 18 or 45. He's either a late bloomer or a premature mess.

I like boys in trouble because I can be both their nurturing Daddy and the Dirty Old Sadist who prods their vulnerabilities. I like weak boys because they make *me* feel stronger, and this way the score is kind of evened-up. It may not seem fair, but it *is* fair. Corey is young, beautiful, and intelligent. My slightly soiled romanticism says that he should be happy, but he's not. It's a mystery, the way all sexual attraction is a mystery, troubling and unfair. How, on the basis of a hesitant smile, elegant profile, and protruding hipbones, have I ended up with an everlasting boner for some thoroughly lost boy? And what, after all, does that say about me?

Sexual need, when you get right down to it, is impossible, illogical, only slightly manageable at the best of times. No wonder religious fundamentalists, set on imposing their tidy schematic plan on the wild and wooly mess that is our world, view sexuality with hostility and mistrust—it just doesn't make sense. And perversion, that moment when my piss was rolling down Corey's lean chest and the heavens opened, perversion makes the least sense of all.

I leave a phone message for Corey wishing him a Merry Christmas. No reply. Same for New Year's.

Eventually, though, I do get Father Bill on the phone.

"Corey left for New York a couple of days ago. He's going to try to get his life together, he said. He's taking the train, should be in Chicago by now."

"The train?"

"His wallet got stolen. Or he lost it. Anyway, no ID, so he couldn't fly."

"New York, huh?"

"His rich Dutch friend is flying over to meet him."

Whatever. Corey, the boy of my dreams, the obsession of my nightmares, is out there somewhere, headed for something. Without identification. And he hadn't even called to say goodbye.

"Allen's still coming around here. He stands outside and yells. Yesterday he demanded to be let in, said he could see Corey through the window."

"Jesus! If you'll excuse the expression."

"I'll miss Corey," the priest says.

"So will I, he's a sweet kid. But fucked-up."

"Yeah," says the priest, "fucked-up."

A few days later I get a pleasant surprise. I come home to a waiting phone message: "Hey, this is Corey. I'm not in San Francisco anymore. I'll call again later."

He's cared enough to phone. I am (maybe pathetically) grateful that I haven't been altogether off-base about him, blinded by my lust, that he really is a nice kid. I figure, however, that he won't actually call again. And he never does.

CHAPTER 16
Pampered: Diaper Play and Other Infantilisms

The pictures he's E-mailed show him lying in a playpen in diapers, hard-on obvious, sucking on a pacifier, surrounded by the signifiers of infancy: baby bottles, toys, a rattle. Goo goo.

Twenty-one. He's 21, which for me is on the cusp of *too* young. He's 21, but he wants to be 6 months old. He warns me he'll want to smoke crack before he plays with me, and let's face it, the only real problem with drug addiction is that it fucks up people's lives, sometimes beyond redemption, so who am I to say no? Right?

After all, lots of things fuck up lives. Lots.

Well, what am I *supposed* to say? I invite him over. Of course.

When he shows up at my door—and he does actually show up at my door—he's as cute as his online pictures, pictures that didn't show the dark circles under his eyes, but I'm used to that, that look of perfect young boys who don't get enough sleep. Not enough sleep. He's considerably more fragile-looking than his power over me would suggest, visibly tweaked but otherwise presentable. My heart, I confess, takes one of its little leaps. Infants are helpless. Crack addicts are helpless. My heart is helpless.

He makes himself at home, nervously. Tweakers talk too much, then apologize for talking too much. I assure them it's all fine. I stroke their drug-blank faces, pull down their pants.

God, he is so beautiful. And he seems intelligent and nice, but then, that's how I want him to be. Sweet and twisted and horny. So that's how he is, then.

Twisted. Fucked-up. Why would a young, beautiful boy want to have sex with someone damn near old enough to be his grandfather? (Funny how the opposite question almost never gets asked. At least by me.) Well, let's look at it another way: Why would someone want to be put into diapers, treated as a child, all the while on a drug-fueled rush?

Because he is, in a phrase, fucked-up. But best not to dwell too much on that, at least not when he's draped across my sofa, the already open fly of his baggy pants thrust forward. He takes off his baseball cap.

My partner? He's at work. I'm not cheating on him; it's a really, really open relationship. He even knows this boy is coming over, though I tastefully haven't shown him the relevant pictures, the way I've sometimes shamelessly done.

My partner, whom I love with all my heart and soul, doesn't want me to remain sexually monogamous with him, no more than I mind when he fucks around with other guys. He wants me to be happy. And he wants me to be safe. I feel the same about him.

Clearly, doing a diaper scene with a young boy on crack doesn't qualify as "safe," at least not in the minds of normal people. Maybe it even squicks *you*, I don't know. I do know that as he reaches into his shoulder bag and pulls out his paraphernalia, assembling the crack bong, heating the bowl, sucking in and puffing out big clouds of demonstrably toxic smoke, I feel like I'm yet again just one horrible step from being a truly predatory old fag, the stuff of right-wing horror tales. I can live with that.

"Oops, my shoe's up against your pillow. You mind?"

I reach down and untie his battered sneaker.

"I'm really sweaty. My feet probably stink. You mind that?"

Quite the opposite. "That's fine," I say, "I'm pretty kinky." Ha ha ha—I'm saying that to a boy who likes to put on a diaper and piss in it. His socks are moist. I bend over and take a sniff. I feel like I'm the luckiest chicken hawk in town.

His cell phone beeps. He takes it. A woman's voice. Though I discreetly leave the room so he can talk, I can tell he's making excuses to her.

"Sorry about that," he says when I get back. "My mom."

Quicksand. "That's OK."

He reaches for the pipe again. I'm starting to suspect that this is one adventure I'm not going to discuss with my partner.

I stand up between his spread legs, my knees pressing out against his thighs. After he's taken the hit, he asks me what's wrong. Nothing, I assure him. And almost nothing is.

"Want some?"

It's been years, many years, since cocaine has entered my system, and I haven't missed it at all. But I don't want to be stand-offish. Nope, I don't want to be left out, not where a cute young guy is concerned. Nope. I sit down beside him. While he heats the bowl, I inhale a smallish hit of the dope.

There's a rush, but it doesn't feel particularly good. After the first few seconds, I just feel edgy. I'm glad, in a way, that I'm not enjoying the coke.

Sober or stoned, I want to see his dick. I reach down to his unzipped crotch. Nice handful. It's easy to undo the drawstring and pull his pants down. He has on black jockstrap-style underwear. I feel the hefty, semicurled shaft through the thin cloth, knowing that this is the moment I'll first see his cock, a moment that, whatever comes later, is never going to be repeated. Undies down. His dick is half-hard and bigger than it has any right to be. And his crotch is shaved; not a surprise, not a turn-on. Just shaved.

He yawns. "I don't know, I'm sleepy, you'd think with all this crack I wouldn't be, huh?" He laughs, then yawns again. I'm playing with his cock and it's getting harder. Christ, I almost never get the chance to suck such pretty young dick. I take it between my lips, fill my mouth with it. A treat. Like full-fat ice cream—delicious, but bad for me at my age. He gets harder, kind of.

"Stop," he says, jumpily. "I'm not really into that. The diaper thing is what I came here for. We talked about that, right? You agreed?"

I take my mouth away. "Sorry," I say.

"Why'd you do that, suck my dick?" he says, as though it were a genuine puzzle, one that pisses him off.

"Jesus. Sorry, OK?"

I tug his shirt up. He doesn't stop me. His lean chest is entirely hairless, his nipples pink and symmetrical and untouched by time.

"You have any stuff?" By "stuff" he means diapers, training pants, baby wipes, talcum powder, baby oil. Well, no.

"I left my things over at a friend's house," he says. "It's not far from here, I'll go get it."

Speed freaks always seem to be between apartments. Their stuff is always at someone else's house. Speed freaks. Crackheads. The things I find on AOL. Jesus.

"We can go buy diapers at Walgreens."

"No problem, I won't be long."

I know damn well what that means. To boys who use illicit central nervous system stimulants, time is flexible. As flexible as morality.

God, 20-something tweakers. I think back to lying in Corey's bed till dawn, waiting for him to return from some meth-drenched errand. Now I want to get this new cracked-out boy in my bed, naked except for a diaper. I want to watch his face as he lets his piss flow, as he wallows in a feeling that goes way the hell back to when he was a newborn. I want to reach down and feel the warm stiffness of his crotch through the plastic diaper, to undo the diaper, open it to the whiff of pee, change him, sprinkle his pretty young butt with sweet-smelling baby powder.

These are things I could never do with my boyfriend, things I could do with, well, nearly no one. I look down at him, lying there with his big dick lolling against a skinny thigh, his scrawny chest rising and falling with each drugged breath. I wonder what he's like when he's sober. I wondered how long it's been since he was. Sober. I'm wondering what the hell has gone wrong in his life, in my life. I'm wondering if I could fuck his ass.

"Where are my shoes?"

I hand them to him, though I want to steal them, throw him out on the street in his sweaty white socks.

"I'll be back soon, less than an hour," he says, pulling himself together. "I really want to do this."

"So do I," I say, and most of me means it. My boyfriend will be out till early evening. Even allowing for delays, the kid might be back with his Pampers and training pants in time for a scene. If he gets back at all.

I maybe can stop him, say "No, really, let's just walk out to buy some diapers." But, like lending Corey my leather jacket, letting Diaperboy go is a test of sorts. Corey had passed that test, but then all he'd had to do was get back to his own messy house, something he'd have done sooner or later regardless. Later, on our subsequent "dates," Corey had passed other tests, and he'd failed a lot too, and he was so thoroughly fucked-up that when he left the country to get the hell away from his speed-freak friends I was happy to see him go, though I figured I'd never touch the flesh of such a beautiful young man again. My partner was glad to see him go too; he always has my best interests at heart.

Boys. Fucked-up boys. This one is disassembling the crack pipe, looking for his cell phone, pulling his baseball cap back over his shock of unruly hair. I look at him, hard, and I can suddenly imagine him in some future, as an adult, much older, less cute, less stoned. I hope he'll get through all this in one piece. I'm too sentimental to qualify as "truly predatory old fag," I guess.

Diaperboy makes for the door, telling me once again that he'll be back soon, that he's "really into this." It might be true, might not. A loose grasp on truth is yet another of the crackhead's dubious charms. My hard-on's fading.

When he's gone I press a button on the CD changer, switching from Radiohead to Led Zeppelin. Something about the levee breaking. Just right. Still edgy from the crack, I read the Sunday paper for a while, then do the dishes. I phone Corey's ex-roommate, leave a message asking if he's heard lately how Corey was doing.

Three-plus hours later, the boy still hasn't returned. I don't know *how* I feel about that.

And I suspect I never will.

That wasn't my first brush with infantilism. It had started many years before, in the days before the Internet so thoroughly transformed the way some of us get laid. I was doing the phone sex lines. I met a man who wanted to be my baby boy. In the blink of an ear, his voice changed from the masculine tones of your basic businessman to a toddler just learning to talk. At first it scared the shit out of me. Because it turned me on.

I had never been turned on sexually by infants, little boys, not even jailbait teens. But here I was doing daddy/boy phone scenes with a guy who was 35 going on 2. Part of me loved the perversity of it, plain and simple—the fact that this was definitely, indisputably Wrong. But there was something else there too, something that fluttered, darkly but promisingly, in the peripheral vision of my desire. A baby bat out of hell.

The relationship went on for months, always by phone. He was in a relationship, he said, with a man who didn't understand this part of him. Well, that's the usual pretext for adultery, sure, but in this case it was easy to believe. And bit by bit I began to truly get into it, having Little Boy Lew come sit on Daddy's lap, playing with his little stiff pee-pee, putting my big man dick into his tight poo-poo hole. Of all the kinkiness in my life, of all the sick and twisted things I've ever done or thought of doing, this was clearly the most over-the-edge difficult to figure out, to accept, to reconcile myself to. Surely child molestation, especially the sexual abuse of an infant, is unforgivable. Yet such is the depth and strength of the taboo that the thought police have not only succeeded in desexualizing childhood but criminalizing, at least for a while, pictures of perfectly obvious adults dressed up as schoolkids for erotic effect. Jesus, I don't find real kids even the least bit sexy. So what the fuck had I gotten myself into?

After a while Lew stopped calling. I filed the whole thing away under "interesting experiences," and though I ended up getting into more daddy/boy play after that, the extended infantilism of Lew's schtick didn't recur. At least not too often.

But every once in a while I'd run across someone, usually online, who was into being a little kid, big time.

The first time I ever actually met a diaper boy it was, well, a little weird. He picked me up in his car and we drove to a deserted street and parked, but by the time he'd unbuttoned his Levi's and revealed the Luvs beneath, I was more than a little put off by his total childishness. He really *was* like a little kid, and that didn't do a thing for me. Unless I could see the contrast, the adult man dropping his defenses and shedding decades, it just wasn't hot for me. I was after infantile, not immature.

Fortunately, the next diaper boy I met, Jody, was a tough little cookie. Around 30, he had a streetwise edge to him, more punkish than playpen. So when he regressed to helpless diaper-clad infant, it was dick-hardening indeed. The very first time he called me "Da-da" I almost came.

It had, in fact, taken months to set up that date with Jody. It had been one of those near-endless online flirtations. "Most guys who contact me," he complained, "aren't really into the diaper thing. They think of it as a freak show they're curious about, or they lead me on just to hear themselves talk."

"Well, I'm into it," I assured him, and finally he did turn up, toy bag in tow. I was glad to see how disreputable he seemed. Sleazy but sweet—just my type. Unlike the sex-related suitcases of most of the men I know, Joe's toy bag was full of kid stuff: diapers, pacifier, rubber training pants, rattle. Even a blankie.

It's not as if I didn't know what I was getting myself into, but the perverse power of the scene was still both hot and unnerving. And sexy and scary are two of my favorite things.

To have an attractive young man pretending to be a baby, to caress his hard cock through a Pamper; it's the kind of thing that confirms the darkest crap from the Moral Majority. Yet it was also, perversely, an incredibly innocent moment, as though the plunge into darkness was not only beautiful but comforting. Pretty highfaluting description of sex with a cute young pervert with a pacifier. "Da-da" indeed.

This was beyond the daddy/boy scenes I'd done before. This was industrial-strength perversion. We played, I took pictures, he peed, I changed him, I took more pictures, he came, he left.

Like many another extreme scene, there was the implicit likelihood, at the moment he walked out the door, that despite the obligatory exchange of phone numbers and "let's do this again"s, that this was a one-off, a trick with no future. He'd gotten what he came for, a scene that he might do only rarely. As usual when I found something new and amazing, I was greedy for more. But, really, what were the chances I'd change Jody's di-dee again?

I wondered, as I straightened up the place (and let's face it, bottoms rarely offer to make the bed), just what he thought of what had happened. More, I wondered who he was.

And I wondered What It All Meant.

I guess it was then I started to think about kink in a way that, for me at least, was new, or at least newish. It wasn't just diaper play, I realized, that was "infantile." It wasn't just daddy/boy play that was a replaying of frozen moments from childhood. In significant ways, most of kink is kid stuff. Punishment scenes? Yes, obviously. Bondage? The thrill of playing cowboys and Indians. Pain play? Well, that was something of a stumper. I'd have to think more about that.

One of the oddest yet most transparent kinks—one I love even though I don't share it—is clinically titled *macrophilia*. Or, as I like to think of it, "guys who jack off to giants." It's daddy/boy play taken to the ultimate, the fantasy of being dominated by a man who's much bigger than you. Twenty times bigger. It's *Gulliver's Travels* rewritten as a stroke story, and it's a fantasy that's surprisingly common.

Since the advent of Photoshop, macrophilia porn has grown by leaps and bounds. (By giant steps, one might say, if one were unregenerate about using obvious puns.) If you know where to look, the Web offers plenty of pics of little naked guys in giants' big, strong hands, or being stepped on by enormous feet, even being popped into colossal mouths. Like I said, kinky, weird to those who don't grasp its allure, and a very, very clear throwback to childhood. Just as "Jack and the Beanstalk" is the story of a rugrat in a world of Adult Threat, macrophilia is a sexed-up version of the fractured fairy tale called "childhood."

Which brings us back to the good old quest for the transcendent. We're talking about jacking off to thoughts of getting picked up—literally—by giants, right? If God is our Father, if every father is God, then what's more obvious than fantasizing about some big fucking guy who could kill you with a single swipe of his enormous paw, could crush you beneath his heel, drown you in his piss—and eroticizing all that? One macrophile I met gets off on thoughts of being eaten by big fellows and zipping through their descending colons like some fleshy water slide. He always manages to pass out of their assholes intact, and if that's not a resurrection myth at least as powerful as what Jehovah's Witnesses peddle, I don't know what is. Still, when the pervert is Photoshopping together his giganto-porn, I doubt he *feels* mythic—images of Saturn devouring his children don't likely pop into his lust-filled brain. But that's a lovely thing about kink: You don't have to understand its archetypal nature to get a stiffy. Like any religious ritual, it works on any number of levels, from the elevated theology of Teilhard de Chardin to an illiterate peasant lighting a candle so a saint will save her child.

When it comes to kid stuff, there's also shaving. Say what you will—it emphasizes gym-built physiques, it makes dicks look bigger—shaving also makes a man look decidedly prepubescent. Actual shaving scenes, in which the top denudes the bottom of his fur, generally have a dom/sub aspect, true. But when I watch a porn video in which humongously adult dicks jut from bodies as hairless as a Hollywood starlet's, the paradox makes me wonder just what's going on.

And then there's "gunge."

Gunge is the increasingly popular pie-in-the-face sport of playing with your food. Bottoms get covered with chocolate pudding, raw eggs, mustard, anything that's gooey and gross, and what's surprising and yet not surprising at all is that some pervs think it's thoroughly hot. A less edgy version of playing with piss and/or shit, gunge takes us back to the high chair and bowls of Gerber baby food. There's the humiliation aspect of the scene, of course, and other overtones as well. A whole subspecies of gunge play requires the gungee to be dressed in a suit and tie while getting mightily messed up. An overthrow of bourgeois respectability? A fucked-up flaunting of the riches of a consumer culture that can afford to waste its food? Or is it, most profoundly, what it most obviously seems to be: the inner infant dragging the male authority of Dad down to its own poo-poo pee-pee level?

When we're little, we're powerless, yet afloat in a world of sensory input and diffuse eroticized delights. Each of us, dumped unceremoniously from amniotic Eden into the cold, cruel world, navigates between the comfort of parental support and the threat of adult powers we only vaguely comprehend. For straight men, each fuck represents a symbolic return to the Source, back to the ol' vagina. Gay men don't have that option. Instead, we reconstruct and try to master these lovely, dimly remembered anxious pleasures through a variety of strategies.

It would be easier, of course, to fence off that part of our consciousness. "Normal" folks desexualize childhood, as though they never played with their pee-pees or enjoyed the delicious feelings of holding in poopie. It's one thing to decry the terrors of genuine child sex abuse. It's another to foment child sex panic—heated fantasies of nursery schools conducting satanic rape rituals and every gay man being a potential molester. It hardly takes a genius to realize that the energy spent on keeping the rigorously repressed out of sight can also be directed outward into fevered witch-hunts. Or that two of the biggest dirty secrets in many folks' consciousness—that they might be less than totally straight, and that when they were kids they had more than a few sexualized nerves in their bodies—can be conflated and externalized into Threat.

One of the hoariest neo-Freudian knocks against homosexuality is that it is, in some sense, a case of arrested development. So I'll try to tread carefully here—not that *heterosexual* men don't whimper at the boots of pro dommes or suck hungrily at their surrogate Mommy's tit. But still…

OK, I'm kind of a Buddhist-Taoist-retired-acidhead. So maybe that's why I love the paradox of ultimate unity. As in: What if the heart of kinky darkness is in fact a shining light as well? What if the journey back to childhood in the playroom is not dysfunctional but a healing journey instead? What if allowing ourselves, as grown men, to be not just bravely transgressive but needily infantile—what if that's *a good thing*?

What if these perversions are our ways of managing not just childhood anxieties best left to psychotherapy, but the deepest squirmy secrets about who we human animals really are and what we need?

The arbiters of civilization have a vested interest in propping it up. The ornery beast of sex gets channeled into legally sanctioned reproduction—the family as a unit of production. Heterosexuality is privileged as "the union of opposites." Queer guys, though, encompass the opposites within. (If I were being *really* esoteric, I'd bring up Ardhanarishvara, the hermaphroditic form of the great Hindu god Shiva. But I won't.)

There's the whole notion of polymorphous perversity too: the idea that infants identify as neither male or female, straight or gay, that there are no borders between "I" and "other," between erotic and not. Sure, for some folks, kink provides an escape, and maybe always not the healthiest one. But what if it's also a strategic retreat to a place we've all been, that we all yearn for? Your own private Eden, though it may look to others like hell.

Kinksters call it "playing" rather than "having sex," not least because the basic genital sex stuff is secondary or nonexistent in many kink scenes. It's a lovely concept, really. That notion of playing—rather than "having sex" or "making love" or, weirdest of all, "sleeping with"—is in itself telling. The childish overtones of the word, the idea that when it comes to sex everything is up for grabs, even the idea that we should have *fun* with our bodies, all runs counter to instrumentalist, late-capitalist civilization and its dick-shrinking dicta. The boringly normative idea of "mature sexuality" equates sex and productivity: Whether love or heirs, fucking should *make* something. But play has no aim but itself.

C'mon, kids, let's play.

CHAPTER 17

Toward a Topography of Desire: Summing Up, Kind of

The other day my friend Bruce said to me, "Isn't life great? Just when you think you've got it all figured out and you can coast till the day you die, you get hit over the head with something new. Big surprises. Everything changes. There's always something to learn." It sounded like Dear Abby, like one of those Maya Angelou Hallmark cards, like a psychobabble show on PBS. But Bruce was talking about kinky sex.

Kyle is 20, well-hung, and—I think—very good-looking in that equivocal way that makes you wonder what 20 more years will bring. He wants older men to wash his mouth out with soap, then forcibly have sex with him. He insists he's not gay—just a "retarded heterosexual." When he was younger, his stepfather used to punish him by making him strip, then washing his mouth out with soap. Kyle found this, he says, strangely erotic, so he didn't mind when his stepdad replaced the soap in Kyle's mouth with his cock. Soon he was servicing a couple of his stepfather's buddies as well. This is what Kyle told me, anyway. Of course, I have no way to know whether any or all of this story is true. But I suspect it might well be. "It's weird," he's said to me. "The right kind of punishment and humiliation makes me feel safe and warm." That seems to be the voice of experience speaking, not something a man just barely out of his teens would invent.

"Did you love your stepfather?"

"Yes," Kyle says.

"And now?"

"I don't live with him anymore. But…yes. I love him. I do."

I'm both appalled and fascinated. And I'd be lying if I said I didn't want to wash Kyle's mouth out with soap. You could think of Kyle's obsession in a number of different ways. As a clear case of arrested development. As a brave making-do. As a surrender to neurosis. As a triumph over abuse or as a capitulation to cruelty. As one more example of the infinite variety of erotic delight or as evidence of a shameful, disgusting crime. And no matter your choice, you'd be right.

One of the beautiful things about kinky sex—maybe the *most* beautiful thing—is its inherent weirdness. We like to pretend that desire is somehow manageable, that it's a game, like Scrabble, we can play and then put back on the shelf. But isn't the hunger for another man—his body, his soul, his cock—the willingness to do so much just to rub up against another animal, isn't that all just an incredible mystery, as boundless as the stars, as never-ending as some sperm-laden sea?

Saint Paul, in his grumpy old body-hating way, set Western civilization on a course from which it's yet to fully recover. He ranted, prune-faced, that sex was no damn good. OK, in a pinch it might just barely be tolerable if it were *for* something: procreation, Christian love within a Christian childbearing marriage. And since then the straight world has taken desire and tried to squeeze it into an itty-bitty box, from which some of its stunted tendrils spring forth, distorted: as wife-beating, as homo hatred, as the religious right's hissy fits.

But let's cop to it. Heaven notwithstanding, sexual desire is just a shitload more strange and more wonderful than any of us can fully comprehend. And kink, which is clearly not progeny-making, which is not bounded by the strictures of "decent" and "reasonable," puts sex squarely back where it's always belonged—in the realm of the magical and senseless and stupid and thoroughly holy.

Queer sex is a complicated beast. We males are competitive and aggressive; it's fuckin' hardwired. It's not just a matter of butch—even the most feline of drag queen carries claws. When two males fuck, the primal struggles for dominance are never far beneath the surface. And yet, and yet…queer male love is about about so many other things too. Including, maybe, transcendence. In the case of kink, a messy transcendence.

Anyone who's been to leather bars, circuit parties, or Palm Springs might find it hard to take seriously the idea of gay men as enlightened *bodhisattvas*. And hey, I find it hard too—like everybody else, most of us queers are unenlightened indeed. What most of us are not, however, is in love with invulnerability. We know the joys of surrender to another man as well as the power that another man's surrender bestows. There's something about getting fucked up the ass that clarifies the mind wonderfully. The desires we have, freed of the reproductive imperative, turn out to be more about distilled pleasure than dynasty-building. We are, despite the proscriptions of society, imbued with a hunger for other men; a hunger that, whatever our enemies might say, truly ennobles. It does not make us less than men. Even the Roman emperor Hadrian, ruler of half the world, was overpowered by his boyfriend's beauty.

Beauty. I admit I'm a sucker for it. A smile, the curve of a leg, the shape of an ear, the face of an angel on Earth, and I'm trapped again, trapped by desire, the impossibilities of loveliness. Yes, it's superficial. Yes, even the most gorgeous boy will someday be dust. And no, not even the Buddha could prevent me from cruising that guy who's pissing at the next urinal. Matter of fact, that dude *is* the Buddha.

OK, so what does this all have to do with getting dressed up in chaps and having the shit beat out of us? Though it would perhaps be reassuring to believe that what happens in the play-room is all just forgettable fun, I can't quite buy that. There's other, deeper, more ornery stuff at stake. So what does the inter-section of power and desire mean to queer folks? And how does it differ, if it does, from the desires of het leather folks?

The rise of international terrorism is said to have "robbed us of our sense of security," but gay men have never felt truly secure. The past decades, despite progress in gay rights and social acceptance of queers, haven't been easy for us. The more visible we become, the more likely we are to be targeted. And though the constant drumbeat of the losses from AIDS have of late become more like tension-filled background noise, the threat of viral doom remains, coiled and ready to strike. Not a few of us have status, wealth, strength, yet I'd wager that buried in even the richest queer CEO's breast is the warning of our fearful history. Those of us who've read our Foucault know that lines of power are never as simple as they appear, but when it comes to the flux between power and powerlessness, we queer men can take com-plexity to head-spinning heights.

How reassuring, then, it might seem to *play* with power. "I'm a big executive," a prospective trick says to me, "so I need to let go and be submissive every once in a while." It's the compensa-tory model of S/M, of course, and pretty much a threadbare cliché. But like many clichés, there's more than a kernel of truth there. And sure enough, when Mr. Big Executive shows up and I put the dog collar on him, he's in hog heaven. We both are. He's come over so I could his fulfill his fantasies of being a groveling bottom, and truth be told, I'm at his service, and that's just fine with me. So the usual question (at least among us who don't take Illusion for Real) arises: *Who's really on top?*

The actual answer is: "We both are." And: "Neither." Both at the same time. Like I said, complex. More complex than some of us, longing for life to have the simplicity of a porn story, would prefer.

OK, here's what I think. I think we all are straining under the burden of mortality, no matter what myths we may construct that promise a happy ending to our earthly lives. As Leonard Cohen, that most Jewish-Buddhist of bards, sings, "We are so small between the stars / So large against the sky." And one way past that heavy load is to use our bodies for pleasure, for con- nectedness, for sex. Orgasm is the quick and dirty way to ego loss, and if it, unlike true enlightenment, lasts but a moment, hey, at least it's always at hand.

S/M play tests the limits of our bodies. Kink butts up against the borders of our souls. How much can we take? How much can give us pleasure? Where are our limits, both as bottoms and tops? As thinking, feeling human beings? In that moment when a bottom's willpower allows him to ask for one more stroke of the whip, when the top makes possible his surrender, there's a dark kind of transcendence. The soul breaks free. And yet it's all about bodies, and physicality reigns over all. Another paradox. Got that?

I think what I'm looking for here is a way out. Every once in a while, some event, whether the lonely death of Matthew Shepard or the deaths of thousands in the Twin Towers, brings me up short. When it comes to S/M, I'm certainly a switch, but one with a wide swath of sadism. How in the hell can I take pleasure in the suffering of another human being, be it ever so circumscribed, consensual, begged-for? What does that say about me?

One answer, of course, is "Shut up and keep flogging." But many of us who've stuck our hands in the fire of kink find that the flames transform. Power-based sex is a hard magic, a steep and dangerous path to self-knowledge. It can, part of me truly believes, be a meditation.

And it can be a weird kind of salvation, or at least expiation, both sinning and seeking forgiveness all tied up in one untidy, dick-hardening package. For all the many, many rotten things that the concept of "sin" has visited on a suffering humanity, a nice, juicy bit of guilt does have its charms. In day-to-day life the kind of sexual guilt most religions dish out can be disturbing, disabling, deadly. But when your dick is stiff, a little sin is good for the soul.

There was that sleazy Italian topboy I played with a few years back. He was the kind of fellow who'd put me in handcuffs and prop his funky sneakers up on my naked body while he was on the phone negotiating a drug deal, which is exactly what he did. But it's not that, nor the fact that post-trick he made me climb out his window to avoid his roommates, that I recall most vividly. It's that he, bless his Italian-American heart, made me recite the Catholic Act of Contrition. That wasn't something the rabbi had taught me for bar mitzvah. Sleaze Boy would recite a line and then I'd repeat it. "Oh my Lord, I am heartily sorry for having offended Thee." Stuff like that. It was a really ripe moment. It was, for a nice Jewish boy like me…um…extremely edifying. (As edifying, I shamefacedly admit, as when abusive Herr Vater curses at me in German.) "Oh my Lord, I am heartily sorry for having offended thee…" As I lay bound and blindfolded on his messy floor, I was filled with the blissful gratitude of the bottom. I felt as blessed as the Blessed Virgin Mary: The expiation of guilt for being alive that religion offers but with orgasms thrown in—could life possibly get any better? Jesus…

Since then, if I'm playing with someone whom I know was raised Catholic, I might throw in a little bit of that old-time religion. I recall a particularly pious evening when I flogged someone who was leaning against a wall, kissing the crucifix he'd hung there. Delightfully baroque. No offense to the many fine members of DignityUSA, the gay Catholic organization locked in constant struggle with the old guard of the Vatican; I'm sure there are many fine and noble things about their religion. It's just that being non-fucked-up about sex isn't one of them.

It's certainly not a stroke of genius to point out how weirdly eroticized Christianity, and particularly Catholicism, looks to the nonbeliever's eye. You're kneeling before this nearly naked guy being tortured on a cross, in pain but also on his way to bliss, and you stick his flesh in your mouth and drink his bodily fluids. Hmmm. Hmmm. Hmmm.

The writings of the ecstatic Saint Teresa of Avila are full of references to being pierced to one's quick by the shaft of the Lord. Apologists will tell us that the eroticism of Teresa's softcore rhapsodies or the tits and ass of The Song of Songs is merely a metaphor for religious transcendence. Fair enough. But what if they have it exactly backwards? What if religious transcendence is actually a metaphor for a good fuck?

While it's fair to say that all religions have an aspect of the erotic about them, even if it's conflicted with a perverse denial of earthly pleasures, it's also true that, say, Hinduism, notwithstanding the guy-fucks-guy's-ass–guy-sucks-off-donkey sculpture on the temples of Khajuraho, lacks the overripe daddy/boy love-and-pain schtick of the Christian mythos. Shiva got pissed off at his son Ganesh and gave him the head of an elephant, but Jehovah loved his son so much that he sent him down to Earth to be tortured and killed, only then to gather the kid back up in Daddy's heavenly embrace. Yeah, I know, Christianity is a metaphor for the general quandary of incarnation in a physical body, but what is sexuality but our way of coping with a physical body that hungers for pleasure, completeness, and release? Anyway, I'd be interested in knowing if non-Christian cultures produce as much daddy/boy desire as does ours. (I sense a Ph.D. thesis here; any of you queer-studies majors are welcome to pursue it.)

Which is not to say that other sects and religions don't also hop aboard that antisex train. Monotheists, from Holy Rollers to Hasids, mullahs to Mormons, are obsessed with the chance that someone somewhere is gonna pop an unauthorized stiffy. Still, anyone who's read the writings of, for instance, Miss Saint Teresa would have to say that Catholicism has its finger rather firmly on the pulse of barely sublimated sexual hysteria.

On the other side of things, though, the more smiley-faced proselytizers of kink too often seem like, well, Unitarians in leather. All sunshine-bright, guilt-free, and having the gol-durn times of their lives. Sure, it may be sweet, but it doesn't cut deep. Let's put the "sin" back in "sincerely twisted" and the "holy" back in "holy shit!"

The first time I spanked someone after the destruction of the World Trade Center, I asked myself whether this meant I would be capable of blowing up "infidels." And the answer, reassuring and definite, came back: nope. Despite all the blurrings, there's a tremendous difference between consensual and nonconsensual uses of power. I think that's one thing about S/M play that so badly disturbs the non-kinky. When society is based on our collective acceptance of power relations, the knowledges that S/M can bestow—that power is a construct, that nothing about domination is ever very simple—might well be seen as a threat to the orders that be. Power relationships in the real world work best when no one concerned, neither the tops nor the bottoms, questions the state of things. Sexual power-play asks the questions, though. It can lead us past the trap of oppositions, into the dark heart of things. Yin. Yang. The union of opposites. Fuck.

Why then, is the "leather community," or at least its more conventional segments, reputedly so much more politically conservative than American queers at large? Yet another paradox. While the consensuality of leathersex may deconstruct the power plays involved, S/M scenes do seem on the surface to celebrate a power-based society. One can be forgiven for walking out of the dungeon thinking that the world consists of those who deserve to dominate and those who need to be restrained. In the world of S/M (and S/M porn), "slaves" are happy folks only too anxious to serve their masters' firm hands. Any outsider would think that leathersex celebrates the trappings and use of power, and sure enough, it does. So what's a nice, progressive, sadistic queer to do?

What, indeed, are the pathways through the topography of desire? Sexuality is an unearthly gumbo, a dreamscape where the part is taken for the whole, the whole dissolves into ecstasy, and everybody has to take a shower afterwards. What may seem to be someone's terra firma—a mind-set where love is the only goal, anonymous sex degrading, and kink a place where there be monsters—may one day seem as quaint as a 16th-century map of the world.

Maps. Place names. Let's not mistake the maps for the terrain. I was recently taken to task by a leatherdaddy for using the words "top" and "bottom" instead of "dom" and "sub." And, in fact, throughout this book that's pretty much what I've done. Sure, in dominance/submission scenes there's a "dom" and a "sub." But applying those terms to the broader range of kink activities seems awfully reductive. "Top" is positional: He's the one with the flogger, the rope, the hand up another's guy's ass. But, as you have no doubt gathered by now, my view of how power's distributed in S/M scenes is somewhat more complicated. In a consensual scene, the power of the "dominant" party is provisional at best. A dominant who honors a submissive's limits—as all good tops do—is both master and servant. Sorry if I'm tweaking anybody's ultra-butch self-image or ruining anyone's fantasies. But reality, I think, is a lot more complicatedly interesting than made-up rules of how things *should* be. There's plenty of dishing about bottoms who "top from below," while I've been accused of doing the opposite, of bottoming from above, a criticism I'll have to fairly cheerfully live with. There, I've said it. Now can't we just get along? Naked? With your mouth on my dick? Sir?

Maps. Place names. Sexual desire is not a stable land. It is, rather, a world we create for ourselves. Queer people, be we kinky or vanilla, create our worlds because we have to. The regular road rules don't apply to us. There's a generally agreed-upon fiction that sexuality is a place we all understand in more or less the same way. But queer sex, and most particularly queer kink, rears up on its hairy hind legs and yells out *Wrong!* Rules, even including the rules of the dungeon, are—whatever their practical usefulness—a barrier to each of us creating his very own private Land of Fuck.

Things change. I was reading parts of this manuscript to Nik, the part about him, his friend Pam, and me at the Folsom Street Fair.

"Pam's a man now," Nik said.

"What?"

"Yeah. Changed his name to Jess. He's living with his boyfriend."

Things change. I'd just been looking over the section on cross-dressing one last time before it went to the publisher when I was visited by the most charming young man—early 20s, smart, leftist, Jewish, cute—who'd brought along some things to play with on our first date. Out of his backpack came a pink see-through thong, black mesh stockings and garter belt, and a silky violet slip. "I want to be pretty for Daddy so Daddy will love me," he said, pulling the stockings over his hairy legs. And he was. He was pretty, so pretty. And somewhere between the rimming and the kissing, me turned totally on by a bearded Daddy's boy in frillies, I realized I'd just have to rethink that stuff I'd written about not getting off on guys in drag.

Things change.

We can not only make up the rules as we go along, we can make up the game. Make up the game board. Make up the world.

Sometimes it seems that desire is not in fact a topography, a navigable landscape we move through, a layer of loamy desire over bedrock. It seems instead a topology, a stretchy surface subject to constant movements, distortions, changes of shape, of focus. It's like being on acid, when everything, the body of flesh, the body of desires, is in fabulous flux. Not one map but many, a dreamscape that shifts with every step.

Hard-core fetishism, far from being a sunspot disturbance in the stratosphere—psychic radio static—can be a stabilizing force, a pushpin stuck through the ever-changing road map. It's the very definition of a fetish: a cathexis of libidinal need. *Whatever happens,* the true fetish says, *you'll need ME to get off.* As Jesus is to Christians the fixed star around which all history turns, the universe of the fetishist spins around the nova of the shoe, the jockstrap, whatever. Stability, be it ever so provisional. It's all well and good to get off when someone drips hot wax on your dick. But if you *need* hot wax to get off, then you'd better have a good-size stock of candles.

The merely kinky, among whom I count myself, don't have the obsessive purity of the fetishist. There's not one focus but a multitude of foci, spicy little ingredients floating in the gumbo of rut. It can get confusing. It can be a challenge to the notion of the unitary self.

On one hand, there's the singular obsession of the True Believer. On the other, postmodernism of the penis. And who the hell knows in which direction salvation truly lies?

I occasionally have phone sex with a 21-year-old in the San Fernando Valley. His voice is so sweet, so innocent. When I asked him if he had a snapshot of himself he could send me, he giggled and said, "My Mom does." Ostentatiously naive. But the things we talk about, the places I take him, the degradations I "force" on him…Jesus, they would have scared the hell out of me at that age. It took a few conversations before I found out that he'd actually once gone to a local park and, after sucking an older man, drank his piss.

"How'd you feel afterwards?" I asked.

"Dirty. I felt good. I don't know," Kev said in that boyish voice of his.

There's nothing, I guess, that excites me in quite the way that sullied innocence does. That is, if you can call a boy who's drunk a stranger's pee, or who jacks off while talking to a stranger about the deepest, most extreme sorts of degradation, "innocent." I choose to think of him that way, though, as a tender, innocent kid. Because part of him is. Just as part of me is still the innocent kid appalled by the thought that anyone could spank someone they love…and get off on it.

"So do you talk about this with anyone else?"

"No, Daddy."

"But you talk about this with me, boy?"

"Yes, Daddy."

"And do you know why, pussyboy?"

"Why, Daddy?"

"Because I understand that the lower you go, the more you want to be my toilet and my cunt, the more ennobled you feel. The freer you become. The more whole you are."

"Oh, Daddy, my dick is so hard."

I, of course, have to strain to keep from coming right then. Eventually, as he repeats, again and again, the degrading things I've told him to say, we do both shoot off. I can hear him catching his breath, then a giggle. I'm wondering if I'm falling in love. I'm wondering who the hell he really is. I'm wondering who the hell *I* am.

"That was amazing," he says sweetly, my sick little pussyboy fag. God, I *am* falling in love.

"Yep," I say—sweetly too, I hope.

"Talk to you soon," Kev says, and hangs up.

Everything changes, the Buddha teaches, and desire is the great snare. So I suppose that phone sex with Kev has guaranteed me at least a dozen more incarnations.

Somewhere in the middle of our conversation, I said to him, "While you're jacking off, I want you to think of this: I want you to think of going in to work tomorrow morning and saying aloud to your coworkers, 'Last night I talked to a stranger about how much I wanted him to shit on me.' "

"Oh my God, oh my God," Kev gurgled. "That's...so...hot."

The good old Cosmic Riddle goes, "Am I a man who sometimes dreams he's a butterfly? Or a butterfly who dreams he's a man?" Is Kev an innocent who fantasizes he's a degraded slut? Or a whoreboy who still fancies he's innocent? When I play Daddy to his boy, am I a wise man pretending to be a monster? Or am I truly a monster only deluding myself that I'm wise?

Has my soul been hijacked? Or is it headed straight toward Paradise?

Oh, Daddy, Daddy, Daddy.

But Even So...

I'm at the gym, and I've just been felt up in the locker room. I'd been putting on my workout clothes when I spotted a man smiling at me from across the room. He looked "interesting" rather than handsome, but his attentions made my dick hard. So I sauntered over to the bench where he sat.

"What's that book?" he asks.

I'm carrying my friend Michelle Tea's *Valencia,* something to keep me occupied as I pedal to nowhere on a stationary bike.

He holds out his hand, just inches from my crotch. "May I see it?" he asks. I hand the book to him. He glances around the locker room, then opens the book so one of his hands is firmly planted against my swelling crotch.

He leafs through the book, discussing literature, groping me all the while. I am struck, not for the first time, by the sheer wonderfulness of being a slut-fag-pervert.

Literature Fan has just gotten dressed and is about to head home. I am, at that moment, more interested in aerobics than in making a date. So when he's finished leafing through the book and fondling my crotch, we hug, surprisingly fondly, and I, still semi-hard beneath my baggy shorts, head up to the workout room.

And there, seated on a stationary bike, is Corey's roommate, Father Bill. My thoroughly stupid heart skips a beat.

"Hey, Bill, you work out here too?"

"Just starting."

I take a deep breath. "You heard from Corey lately?"

"As a matter of fact, I have. His Dutch boyfriend came over to New York to meet him, and they went back to Amsterdam together. Corey's living there now."

"Hey, that's great," I say, and mean it. I really do care about Corey, and I want him to get his tattered life together.

But what if Corey hadn't left town when he did, what then? What if he, if any of the bottomboys I've pursued had fallen for me hard, had wanted to be not just my trick, my spankee, my temporary sub, but my partner? Would I have thrown over my relationship for a kid who, when he got to be my age, would most likely have my ashes on his mantle? Nope, not bloody likely.

And maybe, I think, that's precisely why I choose these dangerous boys—because they're safe. Because, let's face it, they're just *too* cute, *too* kinky, too much fun. There's no way I could ever settle down with one of them without feeling like I was his permanent mercy fuck. There's no way, even in my most weightless moments on the roller coaster of lust, that I could seriously entertain the idea of starting a dangerous new life with a charming, feckless boy—a boy like Corey.

As much as I like my play partners, as easily as I fall in love, I'm either too grounded or too earthbound to base my whole emotional life on someone who gets hard when he calls me "Sir." (Not to mention my utter devotion to my long-suffering present partner.) I respected Corey, I lusted after him fiercely, but at the end of the day, there was no way he could ever be more than a bit on the side. If it's true that nothing brings more sorrow than answered prayers, then by worshiping at the altar of the Blessed Twisted Bottomboy, I more or less ensure that I'll happily go on longing, forever and ever, amen.

More likely—more realistic, of course—is that if Corey had stayed in San Francisco, we would have seen each other occasionally, maybe even regularly, for a while. And then he would have moved on to someone else; or to no one else but away from me; or else I would have realized that whatever I thought he was, could have meant to my life, he was, in reality, not that. And my expecting him to *be* that, whatever it was—Dreamboy, Lost Boy, Deep and True Fuck Buddy, whatever—would have been a burden he couldn't deal with, didn't want. And that would have been that, the usual irresolute ending to grand-but-impossible passions.

When you're young and look at the old folks, you see compromise, disappointment, barely submerged despair, and you think, *That will never be me.* You'll be different, escape the bruises. Remain true to your hopes and ideals. But life has other plans. Life always has other plans.

Sex, death, desire, life, and HIV—it's a messy, unlikely stew. Eat up.

Kink. Fisting, flogging, pain, piss, feet, father/son…if, indeed, the goal and the journey are one, then it's been a helluva trip.

And Corey? I wish he were here so I could stroke his lovely face.

And then slap it. Hard.